# Treating Violence: A Guide to Risk Management in Mental Health

# Treating Violence: A Guide to Risk Management in Mental Health

Tony Maden MD MRCPsych
Professor of Forensic Psychiatry
Imperial College London
and
West London Mental Health NHS Trust

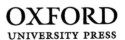

OXFORD
UNIVERSITY PRESS

# OXFORD

UNIVERSITY PRESS

Great Clarendon Street, Oxford OX2 6DP

Oxford University Press is a department of the University of Oxford.
It furthers the University's objective of excellence in research, scholarship,
and education by publishing worldwide in

Oxford New York

Athens Auckland Bangkok Bogotá Buenos Aires Cape Town
Chennai Dar es Salaam Delhi Florence Hong Kong Istanbul Karachi
Kolkata Kuala Lumpur Madrid Melbourne Mexico City Mumbai Nairobi
Paris São Paulo Shanghai Singapore Taipei Tokyo Toronto Warsaw

with associated companies in Berlin Ibadan

Oxford is a registered trade mark of Oxford University Press
in the UK and in certain other countries

Published in the United States
by Oxford University Press Inc., New York

© Oxford University Press, 2007

The moral rights of the author have been asserted

Database right Oxford University Press (maker)

First published 2007

British Library Cataloguing in Publication Data

Data available

Library of Congress Cataloguing in Publication Data

Maden, Tony.
Treating violence : a guide to risk management in mental health / Tony Maden.
  p. ; cm.
Includes bibliographical references and index.
ISBN-13: 978-0-19-852690-2 (alk. paper)
ISBN-10: 0-19-852690-3 (alk. paper)
1. Dangerously mentally ill--Rehabilitation. 2. Violence--Treatment. 3. Mental
health facilities--Risk management. I. Title.
[DNLM: 1. Mentally Ill Persons--psychology. 2. Violence--prevention & control.
3. Mental Disorders--complications. 4. Risk Assessment. 5. Risk Management. WM 600
M181t 2007]
RC569.5.V55M34 2007
616.85′82--dc22                                                    2006033355

ISBN 978-0-19852690-2 (Pbk.)

10 9 8 7 6 5 4 3 2 1

Typeset in Minion
by Cepha Imaging Pvt Ltd, Bangalore, India
Printed in Great Britain
on acid-free paper by
Biddles Ltd., King's Lynn, Norfolk

# Foreword

One of the great fallacies in modern mental health care is that being concerned with risk is essentially anti-patient. Anything you do to reduce risk in mental illness, this argument runs, adds to stigma, reinforcing public prejudice by confirming that mentally ill people may be violent, pandering to stereotypes created by the media.

So it is important to say clearly that most people with mental illness are not violent, and that most violence in society is carried out by people who do not have mental illness. The risk that a member of the general public will be the victim of a random attack by someone who has slipped through the net of community care is very small. And hostile attitudes to the mentally ill are less common in people who have personal experience of mental illness through friends, neighbours and family – in other words, fear of mental illness is more common in people who know little about it.

Even so, it is an undeniable fact that mental illness is associated with an increased risk of violence. It is equally undeniable, however uncomfortable, that there are often failings in the care of mental health patients who carry out serious assaults on others. And when such incidents occur, the consequences are extremely serious for the mentally ill person. More than that, such incidents are in themselves bad for stigma, not least because they reduce public confidence in mental health services.

My concern is therefore that good risk management should be part of routine clinical care, that all frontline services should have the skills to assess and manage risk. In one sense, it does not matter that serious violence by mentally ill people is rare – plane crashes are rare but we expect airlines to do everything they can to improve safety. The response of mental health services should be similar and the result should be better, more comprehensive packages of care for many patients, prevention of catastrophe for a few.

Tony Maden's book tackles these issues head on. This should come as no surprise to anyone who has read his articles or attended his lectures. He is not only a leading authority on forensic mental health but a prominent exponent of structured risk assessment in mental health care, well known for his trenchant views.

His book is not a dry academic treatise. It is a highly entertaining polemic, a personal statement, not just about clinical risk management but about, as he sees it, pseudo-liberal attitudes and the mess they have got us into. Professor Maden argues that structured risk assessment is vital to improving safety in mental health care but he goes well beyond this – dismantling the opposition from RD Laing to his own colleagues. He sets out a history of the strained relationship between services, patients, policy-makers and the public on the issue of risk and mental illness, boldly referring in his opening line to the killing of Jonathan Zito by Christopher Clunis in 1992 as "the most important event in the history of modern British mental health services".

A senior figure in British psychiatry once complained to me that the Department of Health was obsessed with risk – of suicide as well as violence. Can you imagine a specialist in any other branch of medicine taking an equivalent view? I have heard leading psychiatrists claiming on television that the profession is not up to the task of assessing risk and, by implication, protecting the public. Can you imagine what effect this has on public prejudice, public confidence and therefore stigma? People who hold these views may object to Tony Maden's book but they should certainly read it – apart from anything else, it is a very enjoyable performance. But they should pour a stiff drink first.

*National Director for Mental Health*                          Professor Louis Appleby
*Department of Health*

To Kieran, Carla, and Rachel. I hope they
will always find risks worth taking.

# Acknowledgments

I wish I had said that

Oscar Wilde

You will, Oscar, you will

James McNeill Whistler

I could write a book of acknowledgments because I am on the side of Wilde and the magpie. I hear something that appeals this week and next week I am saying it myself. It's a science thing; ideas are useful so long as they help to make sense of the facts, but there is no place for sentimental attachments when a better one comes along. This underlying principle distinguishes medicine from politics, religion, and the law—or at least, it ought to. So I have tried to take something from everyone I have worked for or with, and I am grateful.

Four people stand out. John Gunn taught me how to be a forensic psychiatrist; Paul Mullen has useful things to say on most subjects, psychiatric or not; Louis Appleby has tirelessly promoted the obvious but long neglected notion that the important thing about mental health care is what happens to the recipient; and Steve Hart taught me how to make sense of risk assessment. Their influences run throughout this book but the errors and biases are all mine.

## A note on terminology

This book is concerned with the risk of violence associated with mental disorder. Whenever I speak of risk without making the context clear, I am referring to the risk of violence in association with mental disorder. Mental disorder is associated with other risks, including the risk of suicide, but I make only passing reference to them. That is not because I consider them unimportant, but because I can only do one thing at once.

The book is not concerned with the short-term management of violence and disturbed behaviour, or with techniques such as de-escalation, rapid tranquilisation, restraint and seclusion. They are covered comprehensively by guidance from the National Institute for Clinical Excellence (NICE, 2005). There is a general consensus on the short-term management of violence and this book deals with the more problematic question of managing risk in the medium to long-term.

Most violence is not associated with mental disorder, and I refer at several points to a literature that is concerned with violence risk prediction in general, rather than to the specifics of violence in the context of mental disorder. I introduce this literature, which has grown out of the study of prisoners and other offenders, when it is likely to be of use to the clinician.

Throughout the book I tend to discuss issues in relation to doctors and medicine, although similar comments would apply to mental health workers from any background. I adopt this approach partly out of convenience, but also because the issues involved are conventionally seen as aspects of medical ethics even though they apply equally to nurses, psychologists, social workers, and others working in the field. Many of these allied professions seem to be more aware than doctors of ethical issues in their everyday work, so they should certainly not feel excluded from any discussion framed in these terms.

## A note on statistics

There are none. Well, none more complicated than you would need to put a bet on a horse, which is essentially what you are doing when you manage violence risk. Clinical risk management should not involve elaborate statistics because its focus is the individual and not a population. Just as you do not need to be a breeder or a vet to put a bet on a horse, you do not need to be a statistician to manage violence risk in mental health. In fact, the emphasis on statistics has been damaging to the cause of risk management because it has created an unnecessary mystique. I suspect many clinicians turn over and go to sleep when they hear talk of Receiver Operating Characteristics or the Area Under the Curve—words that are mere foreplay to the statistician—so this is the last time I will mention them.

# Contents

# Chapter 1

# Why worry about violence risk assessment?

The most important event in the history of modern British mental health services occurred on the platform of Finsbury Park tube (subway) station where, on the afternoon of 17 December 1992, Christopher Clunis killed Jonathan Zito. Clunis was a young man with chronic schizophrenia and a history of violence. Jonathan Zito was a young musician, recently married and waiting for a train with his brother when Clunis stabbed him in the face in an unprovoked attack.

There had been many previous homicides by mentally ill people, some of which were followed by independent Inquiries, but the Clunis case became synonymous with the problem. The reasons for its notoriety include the unstinting efforts of Jonathan's widow Jayne to ensure there was a proper Inquiry into the killing, and that action was taken to reduce the frequency of such incidents. There was also the horrific nature of the attack, which came out of the blue, in the afternoon, on an ordinary station platform. But the main reason for the case's infamy was the gross inadequacy of the mental health care given to Clunis in the years leading up to the attack. There was little attempt to assess or manage the violence risk he posed. On the contrary, it seemed the risk was wilfully ignored. Worse still, most of the failings were not due to incompetent or negligent individuals. This was how the system operated. The outcome was unusual but many of the practices were common.

The subsequent Inquiry (Ritchie *et al.*, 1994) was one of the most critical of services and it is still widely quoted. It led to the introduction of new procedures for managing mentally ill people in the community. It led also to the system of mandatory independent Inquiries in England and Wales whenever a person receiving mental health care committed a homicide.

The Clunis case forced UK mental health services to give proper attention to violence risk for the first time. The shape of services changed and violence risk assessment became a central concern. Discussions of violence feature in many if not most care planning meetings, and they probably occur almost as frequently outside work. Whenever and wherever inner-city mental health workers meet, the conversation often touches on violence, whether it is an incident within the service or a homicide Inquiry that has hit the national headlines. A recurring theme of these conversations is the horror of being caught up in an Inquiry, and the unfairness of one's work being scrutinized through the distorting lens of hindsight. People are worried.

Worrying about a subject is not the same as dealing with it. The killing of Jonathan Zito took place over 15 years ago but there is still argument about how best to carry out violence risk assessment—or whether we should do it at all. Some professionals are opposed in principle, and others believe useful risk assessment is impossible in practice. Hospitals have had violence risk assessment policies thrust upon them by the fear of litigation, but most have no clear or systematic rationale and amount to a list of boxes to be ticked. The standard UK approach to violence risk assessment appears primitive alongside examples of best practice, or even routine practice, in countries such as Canada. Yet, as the horror of the Clunis case shows, there can be no higher priority than minimizing the occurrence of this most negative of all negative outcomes.

Services with inadequate procedures for managing violence risk let down patients, relations and carers, as well as potential victims. They also let down their staff. The world is no longer a forgiving place for professionals when things go wrong. If the world is a jungle, or a swamp inhabited by ravenous tabloids, mental health workers deserve better than to be sent into it with their eyes closed.

Some mental health disasters cannot be prevented but many can, and the inevitability of serious violence is an argument for better risk management. Even when the outcome is bad, it is better to know that risks were considered rather than ignored. It is never pleasant to face an Inquiry after a homicide, but it is worse if risks were not recognized when they are obvious from a reading of the records. In simple terms, it is better for the service to recognize risks before a disaster than to have them pointed out afterwards.

So this book is not a neutral, scholarly review. It is a sales pitch for violence risk assessment. It is a prod with a sharp stick for those who argue we should not worry too much about violence by the mentally ill because it is uncommon. It is an argument for better mental health services, meaning better care for patients and better protection for staff. It is a plea for staff to open their eyes, and to get some training before stepping on to the tightrope.

The book is not a systematic review of the literature. I feel under no obligation to include mention of everything ever written on the subject. I include studies if they help to make the point that we can and should have better violence risk assessment. I have left out some good studies because of lack of space, or because they restated a point that had already been made. I have tried not to leave out anything simply because I did not agree with its conclusions; there is no need, because the arguments against a more systematic approach to violence risk management are so weak. Bring them on, as George Bush regretted saying.

I have tried to address the main issues in risk management but not the small print—except when the small print is interesting or essential. References for further reading are given when appropriate. I would love readers to come away from this book with a determination to learn about and use the HCR20 (Historical Clinical Risk-20) or another method of structured clinical assessment, but I would be content if they were simply converted to the view that violence risk management is a good thing that can be done better.

The book grew out of my experience of giving lectures and seminars on the topic of managing violence risk. Some of the lectures were general accounts of the field. Some of the seminars were instructions on using risk assessment instruments and particularly the HCR20 (see Chapter 6). The audiences were from various professional disciplines and the services in which they worked covered the spectrum from high security to community. Some were from prison or probation rather than mental health services, and some were civil servants who never got closer to a violent patient than reading his file.

Audiences have opinions and teaching is a two-way process, so I have made use of feedback and questions that reflect a broad spectrum of viewpoints. Overall, there were more positive than negative responses to the idea of violence risk assessment, but counting the votes misses the point. If you work in mental health, violence risk assessment is up there with death and taxes as one of life's certainties. You can choose to love it or hate it, but you cannot avoid it. And if you have to do it anyway, why not do it well? But, first, we should consider the opposition.

## The Luddite perspective

*Luddites*: A group of men whose object, from about 1811 to 1816, was to destroy machinery used in the developing textile industry. The term has come to be used to designate people who stand in the way of progress, particularly when that progress threatens their own position.

What psychiatry, an essentially medical discipline, has got to do with risk reduction and reducing recidivism remains firmly beyond me …

Sarkar (2003; a consultant working in a high security forensic hospital)

I am persuaded by the arguments in favour of good violence risk management and would be happy to get on and look at how it can be improved. But even the most rabid enthusiast for risk assessment cannot ignore the scepticism still surrounding it, particularly in the UK. The essence of the sceptical view is that violence risk assessment is wrong in principle and impossible in practice. According to this argument, violence risk prediction is no better than chance. Any attempt to assess violence risk will lead to locking up too many people, and the wrong people. At the same time it will stigmatize all who are, or ever have been, mentally ill. Instead of forcing risk assessment on them we should let well-meaning clinicians get on with their jobs and, if things go wrong, shrug and comfort ourselves with the reassuring thought that disasters do not happen often.

These views are, in a word, wrong. Even so, they are common enough to warrant a more closely argued response. For that reason, the first chapter of this book addresses the question: Why worry about violence risk assessment?

I should apologise at this point to those readers who already have their own answers to this question. A double apology is necessary for readers from parts of the world where structured risk assessment has been routine for some years. The fact remains that there are still plenty of mental health workers who believe a book on violence risk management to be unnecessary, misguided, and damaging. Those who are already convinced of the case for violence risk assessment may skip ahead to Chapter 2. Alternatively, the following may provide useful ammunition for the next time you find yourself in a dark alley with a member of the Luddite tendency.

## The case against violence risk assessment
### Medical ethics

The ethical argument against violence risk assessment starts from the premise that, as doctors, psychiatrists have as their main function the relief of suffering. It follows that the doctor's primary responsibility is to the patient, with any additional obligation to society coming a long way behind in second place. The assessment of risk to third parties is therefore low on the list of things a doctor needs to worry about.

This child's view of medical ethics would be strained even in a quiet medical backwater. It is next to useless as a guide to dealing with the dilemmas faced by anyone working in the moral and political war zone of modern mental health services, where doctors comment routinely on issues that go beyond the doctor–patient relationship, and beyond therapy. Psychiatrists give opinions in childcare proceedings on an adult's ability to function as a parent. The doctor's dealings with the adult are based on the explicit principle that his or her needs are less important than those of the child.

If the war zone analogy seems too extreme, consider the emotions surrounding cases in this field. Professor Roy Meadow, a paediatrician, gave (inaccurate) expert evidence that contributed to the wrongful conviction of a mother for killing her children. In due course, the General Medical Council ordered that Meadow's name be struck off the medical register, only for the High Court to overturn that decision on appeal. Their judgment was that the medical expert, giving evidence in good faith, is accountable only to the Court and not to any professional body. Not only may the doctor go beyond any narrow responsibility to a patient, he is under an obligation to do so and is granted special privileges and protection in this task.

This is a world away from the bank robber seeking treatment for his bullet wounds, safe in the knowledge that he is protected by the doctor's Hippocratic Oath. At the risk of robbing people of their illusions, we need to accept that scenario was part of a film; it was a fiction, a story made up for money. Confidentiality and a commitment to the patient's welfare are central tenets of medicine but they have always had their limits.

In the real world a doctor's job was always more complicated than in the fiction—and less exciting most of the time. In all branches of medicine, doctors sign forms to regulate access to sickness or disability benefits, or to pensions. These are mundane examples of medical involvement in the complicated processes of rationing and social control. In all these functions, the doctor's obligations extend way beyond the doctor-patient relationship, and she is often serving at least two masters. Foucault was right, at least in this respect.

Psychiatrists are unusual but not unique within medicine, in dealing with risk to third parties. The best analogy is with the control of infections, where the state has powers to detain patients who may spread a disease. Tuberculosis is the classical example but the outbreak of severe acute respiratory syndrome (SARS) in 2003, with immediate calls for powers to detain suspected carriers of the virus, provided a reminder that these powers remain important.

When we recall that it led to the brief but almost complete isolation of Toronto from the rest of the world, the SARS outbreak is also useful as a reminder of our low tolerance of third party risks associated with medical conditions. The measures to combat bovine spongiform encephalopathy (BSE) in the UK are another good example, in which the livelihoods of many farmers were sacrificed to the greater good. Before that there was *Salmonella* in poultry.

The common theme of these examples is that individuals may ignore medical advice affecting their own health, and we defend our right to smoke or drink ourselves to death, but we do not hesitate to intervene when others are at risk. Hence, many countries have now banned smoking in public places, even though the risks of passive smoking are relatively small.

Similar principles are bound to apply in mental health. If violence to others is occasionally caused by mental illness, which is no longer in doubt (see Chapter 2), then mental health services have to take that risk seriously.

In this context the argument about the risk of suicide grossly exceeding that of homicide appears weak or irrelevant. Most people see suicide in a simplistic way as a risk run by the patient, ignoring secondary victims of the act. It is quite different from homicide, where the risk is run by others. As Tidmarsh (1997) and others have noted, we are particularly averse to risks over which we have no control.

An ethical view of compulsory treatment in order to control violence risk assumes that our patients share these views of acceptable and unacceptable risks, except when their mental state is disturbed by illness. As we are all potential patients, it is a reasonable ethical exercise to ask ourselves about the extent to which we would be willing to put others at risk if we became mentally ill. Although not a cheerful subject to consider, most of us probably find it easier to contemplate suicide while mentally ill, rather than killing or harming a loved one. Is it paternalistic to assume patients share our sense of priorities? Reasoning of this sort underpins the concept of advance directives, and it suggests there may not be so much conflict between social and individual interests when it comes to violence risk. Would any of us want to be allowed to harm somebody when mentally ill?

Ethical reasoning is enshrined in mental health practice by the Tarasoff case (Tarasoff v. Regents of the University of California, 1976). A Californian therapist became aware of a specific risk to a third party who was later killed by his patient. The therapist was held to be negligent in not informing the victim of the risk, the court concluding there was a duty to warn in these circumstances, overriding the normal duty of confidentiality.

In summary, there is a strong ethical case, with countless precedents, for a health professional to act against an individual patient's wishes in order to manage the risk of violence associated with a mental disorder. A single-minded emphasis on the doctor's obligation to the patient alone owes more to fictional or romantic notions than to the reality of medical practice, and it is unsuited to any case in which there is risk to a third party. Finally, it conflicts with the way in which we practise psychiatry at the moment. Most of us who work in adult mental health have been involved in the detention of patients in order to protect other people. We hope that, in taking this action, we are also acting in the patient's longer-term interest but the immediate reason for detention is the safety of others. We recognize the customer is not always right, and so we manage violence risk.

## Capacity and consent

> When you're making your bed, remember you'll do the lying there. When you butter your bread, don't expect me to eat your share.
>
> Your Red Wagon, Mose Allison

Some people accept that we devote a lot of energy to risk assessment and management at the moment, but they argue that our approach is wrong because it discriminates against the mentally ill. They claim we should treat mental disorders in the same way as physical disorders, so there is no need for specific mental health legislation. Treatment would be voluntary in the vast majority of cases, as it is at the moment, and the only reason for intervening without a patient's consent would be if the patient lacked the capacity to give informed consent (Dawson and Szmukler, 2006).

There are many attractions to the capacity-based approach to involuntary treatment, particularly for those who work in mental health. A system based on capacity limits the duty of care owed by a service to its patients. If the patient has the capacity to decide whether or not to accept treatment, then the question of risk does not arise in the assessment for compulsory treatment. More importantly, it will never arise in those patients who choose not to accept treatment. They accept responsibility for all that follows from their rejection of help, so they relieve the service of that responsibility.

It is easy to understand the growing appeal of this notion over the last 15 years, as pressure on services has mounted following a series of critical Inquiries into homicides by patients with mental illness. Capacity-based legislation would turn down the heat in a kitchen that is too hot for many people working in mental health. It also appeals to service users and patients because it respects their autonomy.

The appeal to politicians and the public is less obvious. As noted above, society has a low tolerance for third party risk associated with mental disorder. Inquiries such as the Ritchie report on the Care and Treatment of Christopher Clunis portrayed a mental health service whose desire to unload responsibility had already crossed the border into frank irresponsibility. It was not going to be easy to sell the notion that the powers and duties of the service should be further restricted. Any attempt to relegate risk to second place, behind capacity, was unlikely to be politically acceptable. It was therefore no surprise, or at least no surprise to anyone outside the capacity lobby, when the UK Government rejected the suggestion of the Richardson committee that reforms to English mental health law should be capacity-based (Winterton, 2004). The Government's preferred option was for a system in which risk was the first priority.

The choice was a straightforward political one, between competing priorities and values. Politicians are elected to take such decisions and there are no signs to suggest they found this one a difficult choice, or that they are considering a change of mind. If any doubts did emerge, a brief reading of the headlines concerning the latest homicide by a psychiatric patient would lay them to rest. The suggestion that capacity should be the first and foremost concern in mental health law is politically dead in the UK. Still, it is worth considering its merits, even if only to understand why it was rejected.

The first problem is that mental disorders are different. The prevalence of schizophrenia in the general population of England and Wales is 1% but in people convicted of homicide it is 5% (Shaw *et al.*, 2006) and it is impossible to envisage comparable figures for any physical disease. Unlike broken limbs or heart disease, serious mental illnesses routinely impair a person's sense of values and morality and in a minority that impairment is catastrophic. A mentally ill person may retain capacity even when mental illness has upset the order of priorities that ruled their life when well. The notion of capacity is complicated and raises the question of advance directives or similar devices for protecting patients from what amounts to a change of mind or judgement, brought about by a pathological process.

A second problem is that most psychiatrists are not used to assessing capacity, and it is less easy to define than it first seems. A suggested operational definition, sometimes known as a functional approach to the assessment of capacity, has three components:

i. The patient must be able to understand information about the proposed treatment.
ii. The patient must be capable of retaining and believing that information.
iii. The patient must be capable of weighing up that information and making a free choice.

*Law Reports* (Re C, 1994)

The relationship between these criteria and the severity of mental disorder may be complicated. For example, a patient with pervasive delusions may retain capacity, provided the delusions do not impinge on these three areas. Another patient, with delusions limited to odd beliefs about medication, could lack capacity while most other areas of life remain unaffected.

A third problem is that all these judgements are matters of degree, as few patients will have a perfect understanding of the pros and cons of suggested treatments. It has been established through case law that the test for lack of capacity should be more or less stringent, according to the importance of the decision. Which makes sense; the capacity to consent to having one's toenails cut is not the same as the capacity to consent to amputation of a limb. When considering consent to treatment we need to consider the consequences of the decision, and to err on the side of caution when those consequences are serious.

Applying similar principles to psychiatry, we rapidly get round the circle and back to the barrier of risk assessment. If a person's mental disorder presents a serious risk to others, we should apply a stricter test for capacity. However, we cannot know what test we should apply, without knowing the size of the risk. Capacity-based mental health legislation would leave mental health workers in the same position, of having to improve their risk assessment skills.

A fourth problem with capacity is that it varies over time. The medical paradigm generally involves acute, one-off decisions. For example, the patient must decide on the amputation of a gangrenous leg, or whether to accept a blood transfusion. Capacity is assessed at the point of crisis, a decision is made, and the matter is resolved. By contrast, the controversial decisions in psychiatry involve chronic, fluctuating conditions. Psychotic mental illnesses such as schizophrenia persist for many years, yet the mental state may change from day to day, or even from hour to hour. Mogg and Bartlett (2005) discuss these issues in relation to the question of consent to physical treatment but have little reassurance to offer, part of their advice being to involve the courts at an early stage. If consent to physical treatment is so difficult that only a court can resolve it, what chance do doctors have when the situation is complicated by the introduction of risk to others?

Variation over time also raises the question of how to deal with conflicting measures of capacity at different times. Capacity today is no guarantee of capacity tomorrow. A patient who has capacity in the clinic may have lost it by the time he gets home. With or without the involvement of the courts, this emphasis on the here and now is no basis on which to manage the risk of serious violence in mental illness.

The fifth problem with capacity is the mismatch between ideals and reality. Lawyers love capacity. It lends itself to ringing courtroom oratory about man born free, sovereign over his own body and with the fundamental right to protect it from unwanted intrusion in the name of medicine, just as he is entitled to protection from violence on the public highway or in the public house, etc., etc. This is entertaining in its place, but it is all so middle class. In the messy, dirty, real world the rhetoric sounds hollow. Is mental illness really like physical illness? When did you last come across a group of homeless diabetics or hypertensives begging at your local station? Is it just coincidence, or exercise of freedom of choice, that leads so many street people to spend their day talking to the voices? Are we untroubled that the prevalence of schizophrenia in perpetrators of homicide is five times its prevalence in the general population?

Capacity appeals to people who spend more time in the courtroom or lecture theatre than on the street. Many of the long-term mentally ill are stuck in the revolving door of prison, poverty, and homelessness. There is a cynical and uncaring aspect to the simple application of a capacity test to people in this group, who have limited opportunities to exercise their fundamental rights at the best of times. The message of the capacity test is that those who decide against treatment have made their beds and now have to lie on them. Proponents of capacity criticize the alternative as paternalistic, but there are worse faults than paternalism when working with patients who often have difficulty looking after themselves. Fathers get an unjustly bad press.

Did Clunis have capacity? Sometimes he did and sometimes he did not. Or, worse still, some doctors would say he did, and some would say he did not. One interpretation of the Clunis case (Ritchie et al., 1994) is that services repeatedly brought the patient to the point at which he had capacity then discharged him and left him to sink or swim. Yet it was obvious his capacity would not be retained for long, once prescribed medication was stopped and he was again facing the stresses of life outside hospital.

The Clunis case is discussed in more detail in Chapter 3. For now it is sufficient to note that it shows the capacity test has a sinister side, as a cloak for unacceptable and uncaring professional practice. In the chronically mentally ill, reliance on capacity alone is unsatisfactory because its focus and time frame are too narrow. While Clunis's mental capacity may have changed frequently, a risk assessment would have shown he had difficulty meeting his basic needs, and posed a serious risk of violence to others, for much of the time. A narrow vision of capacity is no substitute for an holistic view, and we have to wonder if the capacity test is serving the interests of professionals rather than patient, if it allows an easy way out when faced by a difficult patient.

Which brings us neatly to the problem of personality disorder. Psychopathy is discussed at some length in Chapter 5, but we should note in passing that a patient with a severe personality disorder may have no difficulty in understanding, retaining, believing, and weighing up information about treatment. Yet his decision may be influenced by psychopathology that attaches more importance to his own convenience than to the suffering of others. Irresponsibility and entitlement are features of psychopathy, and any attempt to assess mental incapacity in that condition is bound to be complicated by questions of risk.

## An impossible task?

I know that half of my patients don't need to be here. Unfortunately, I don't know which half

Apocryphal, but attributed to a former medical superintendent of Broadmoor high security hospital.

According to this model, it is impossible to predict violence so there is no point in trying. A variant on this objection to risk assessment is that doctors have no particular expertise in the field, so it is unreasonable for them to be involved. This view of the world suggests that violence by psychiatric patients occurs more or less at random, so it is pointless to try to guess where it will next arise. The job of the doctor is to get on with treatment and the relief of suffering, and futile attempts at prediction are nothing more than a distraction.

The next chapter considers research on risk in more detail, but it is fair to summarize present evidence as indicating that clinical risk assessment is consistently more accurate than chance. Of course, that does not mean it is possible to predict with any certainty which patients will be violent and when, but it is possible to make reasonable statements of probability. More importantly, it is possible to say what factors will increase or decrease the risk of violence, which is the first step in managing the risk.

Expectations need to be realistic. A favourite tactic of critics is to set an impossibly high standard for risk assessment, then to jettison the whole enterprise when it fails the test. A search for specific predictions is bound to lead to disappointment. Crystal balls do not work, and in most branches of medicine we do not expect them to work. Doctors are content to identify risk factors for complications of various conditions, and we do not criticize the cardiologist for failing to predict which one of his hypertensives will be the next to suffer a stroke.

Even without a detailed consideration of the research evidence, clinical experience suggests that doctors have some skills in risk prediction. Some acts of violence by patients are unexpected and some cases of schizophrenia present with an act of serious violence, but it is still true that previous violence is one of the best predictors of future violence. Psychotic relapses are often similar over time in the same patient, and staff on the intensive care ward know only too well that patients who have been violent during previous admissions will present a high risk of violence in the future. Many of the homicide Inquiries (see Chapter 3) make a convincing case for the presence of obvious risk factors preceding the offence. It is relatively rare for the event to come out of the blue.

It would be disastrous for violence risk prediction if most violence were truly random, but it is not. Violence risk assessment may not be an exact science, but the probabilities involved are on a par with those used in other areas of medicine. In the next section, we consider whether the inevitable uncertainties of this system lead to so many errors that it is not clinically useful.

## False positives and false negatives: the necessity of getting it wrong

It's the economy, stupid

Bill Clinton, on the key to winning elections

Risk assessment has been characterized as the labelling of some patients as high risk and others as low risk. This is a gross oversimplification, and later chapters emphasize the multi-faceted nature of risk assessment. Still, it can be a useful oversimplification. It allows us to consider the technical aspects of risk screening alongside other medical screening techniques, or non-medical procedures.

A good example of an established screening technique is mammography for early breast cancer. Women who rate as high risk on mammography consist of two groups, true and false positives. True positives are the patients who have cancer in its early stages. False positives will turn out not to have cancer.

In violence risk assessment true positives are those who, without intervention, will go on to behave violently. False positives are patients who are rated high risk but will not behave violently. In patients rated as low risk, some will be true negatives but others will be false negatives who go on to behave violently. Any test has two types of errors, false positives and false negatives.

The way we talk about such errors comes from Signal Detection Theory, which was developed during the Second World War to assist in the training of radar operators. As part of Britain's air defence system these operators sat for hours staring at a screen and waiting for a blip to appear on it. A blip was an enemy bomber, leading to an urgent call to scramble the fighters. Except that sometimes a blip was interference or a flock of birds, leading to fighters confronting seagulls. That was the radar operator's false positive and it was embarrassing. However, it was probably less embarrassing and certainly less deadly, than a false negative in which a bomber was ignored in the mistaken belief it was a bird.

The aim of training and improvements in technology was to increase sensitivity; that is, to minimize the number of false negatives while keeping down the number of false positives. The false positive rate is the specificity of a test, and there is an inevitable trade-off between sensitivity and specificity.

We use the terminology of Signal Detection Theory to discuss violence risk assessment but it is a mistake to apply the radar model too literally. It should

**Table 1.1** False positives and false negatives in violence risk prediction

|  | **Actual violence** | **Actual non-violence** |
|---|---|---|
| Predicted violence | True positives | False positives |
| Predicted non-violence | False negatives | True negatives |

perhaps be unnecessary to spell out the differences between a modern mental health service and the Battle of Britain, but here are a few of them.

First, the radar operator is faced by a one-off, all-or-nothing decision. It is either a bomber and you scramble the fighters; or it isn't and you don't. By contrast, violence risk management often consists of a series of smaller decisions—to increase or decrease medication, to mention an observation to a family member, to request an extra appointment, or to allow a move from a staffed to an unstaffed hostel. Feedback from the results of one action affects the next decision, and so on. This chain of decisions is difficult to study. Try applying Signal Detection Theory to the question of whether to increase depot medication, which depends on information from different sources and times, and where the outcome may be impossible to determine. As a result of this problem we tend to concentrate on the big decisions, such as discharge or detention, which distorts the debate about risk management.

Second, the objectives of risk assessment in mental health are less clearly defined than those of a wartime radar station, and the values are different. We cannot prevent all violence by patients, and we need to concentrate on that violence that is most directly linked to mental disorder. One of the central themes of this book is that not all acts of violence are equal, and we have to attach different values to the prevention of different acts.

The question of values brings us to the third difference, which is the acceptability of error. The two types of errors, false positives and false negatives, are important in many fields of medicine. In cancer screening they cause unnecessary anxiety to patients who do not have the disease (false positives), and delays in treatment of some patients who do have the disease (false negatives). In violence risk prediction, patients may face unnecessary detention or unnecessary, compulsory treatment. Some critics suggest the high false positive rates of many violence prediction instruments should lead us to abandon the whole exercise of risk management, but this argument ignores the different values attached to different errors. In order to appreciate the problem, we need first to consider the figures.

There is no easy way around the statistical problem. If it were possible to measure violence risk accurately in numerical terms (and it is not, as will be made clear in later chapters) we may decide to intervene at, say, a 50% or a 10% probability of violence. It is the nature of statistics that, if we adopt the

50% threshold for detaining patients, we would be intervening unnecessarily in half of all patients. With the 10% threshold, nine of every 10 detentions would be unnecessary on average (if 10 people each have a 10% probability of doing something, you would expect only one to actually do it. Even this is an abstraction, which assumes the experiment is repeated an infinite number of times with an infinite number of groups of 10).

These numbers look terrible in terms of cost, let alone human rights. The missing ingredient is the value we attach to preventing a particular error. For the radar operator, a very high value was attached to missing a bomber (avoiding a false negative), so the system tolerated the cost of false positives in order to be sure that true positives were not missed. In mental health we are prepared to impose compulsory treatment, knowing there will be a high rate of false positives, when we are managing serious risks such as life-threatening assaults. The values we attach to different outcomes suggest the price is worth paying.

A fourth fact to bear in mind is that the lessons of Signal Detection Theory apply equally well to unstructured, clinical decisions as to structured risk assessments. Critics present the statistics on false positives as evidence against any form of structured risk assessment, but the same ammunition can and should be used against the easier target of unstructured decision-making. There is no absolute certainty in clinical medicine. High error rates are an argument against any decision-making. They are an argument for inertia, an argument for the armchair philosopher who sees the possible downside of action so does nothing.

Monahan (1981) has pointed out that if you want to be right most of the time, the correct strategy is to predict that no patients will be violent. He also points out the unacceptable nature of this suggestion, because not all errors are equal. The cost of worrying some patients unnecessarily has to be set against the value of saving lives through early detection of cancer, and the same argument applies to violence risk management. This issue is discussed in more detail in Chapter 2, but the simple message is that people who cannot stand the thought of being wrong a lot of the time should probably not go into medicine, and certainly not into the field of mental health.

If the problem of false positives were a fatal flaw, incompatible with ethical practice, doctors would never detain patients because of violence risk. We can never be certain of the future, so any system must inevitably lead to the detention of people who would not have behaved violently if left alone. Yet most doctors are prepared to carry out assessments for detention under the Mental Health Act, using clinical criteria alone. It is the height of medical arrogance to claim that, using only their clinical intuition, they never detain any 'false positives' on the grounds of risk.

This point is important enough to risk labouring it by retelling an old joke. A man approaches a woman sitting at a bar and asks her if she would sleep with him for a million dollars. After brief reflection she says yes, at which point he tells her he does not have a million dollars, so will she sleep with him for fifty? 'Certainly not, what do think I am?' 'Lady, we've already established what you are, we're just haggling about the price.' In other words, the only pure position is to opt out. If psychiatrists are prepared ever to detain a patient on the grounds of risk to others, we know what they are and it is time for some hard bargaining over the price. At the risk of flogging the metaphor to death, is it too much to suggest that standardization of the process of risk assessment is just familiarity with the market? And that only a fool bargains without being aware of the going rate?

There is no way of escaping this issue within medicine, let alone within psychiatry. A change of specialty only translates the problem to a different area. All binary decisions (to treat, to operate, to give a diagnosis, etc.) are subject to similar reasoning, even if we like to pretend otherwise. The only escape is in the delusion that one knows the answer for certain, so fooling oneself as well as the patient. It is much more honest to acknowledge the uncertainty, to work to minimize it, and then to be open about the limitations of one's knowledge. All of which is much easier to achieve by a process of structured risk assessment, which allows us to describe risk in a way that is easily communicated to others.

The final reason for being cautious about applying Signal Detection Theory to violence risk assessment is also the saving grace for mental health and the whole medical enterprise. Unlike radar operators, we can turn positives into negatives—not always, but often enough to make it worthwhile. Treatment makes a difference. An enemy bomber will never turn into a flock of birds, but a patient with proper treatment and support in the community is transformed from an unacceptable risk to an acceptable one. With apologies to Mr Clinton: 'It's the treatment, stupid'.

## The case for violence risk management

To some extent I made this case while rebutting opposing arguments in the previous section, so I deal with it briefly at this point. Also, the question of why we should assess risk deserves a brief answer. We measure because we aspire to be scientific, and science begins with measurement. Measure or die, as Newton and Einstein would have said. Abandon that principle and we throw in our lot with complementary therapists, lawyers, politicians, and others whose output is judged by ephemeral standards.

## The epidemiology of violence and mental disorder

For many years until the 1980s, the orthodox teaching within psychiatry was that there was no link between violence and mental disorder. This period has been described by Tidmarsh (1997) and others as the mythical golden age of psychiatry, when it was not necessary to worry too much about violence risk.

Looking back, it is difficult to understand how this belief was sustained in the face of evidence to the contrary. Anyone working in acute mental health would see people who became violent only when mentally ill. Many staff would have been hit by a patient and most would have been threatened, often by patients with whom they had a good relationship in between periods of relapse. Psychiatric intensive care units trained their staff in the management of aggression, long before it became necessary in other parts of the health service. Was this all just the result of coincidence?

The simple explanation was that the research had not been done. Chapter 2 deals with the development of research in the area, and the main study is outlined below. Even so, while lack of research evidence was a problem, it seems insufficient to account for such gross denial. For many years hospital staff would go from a ward where patients were routinely violent or threatening in response to psychotic symptoms, to a lecture theatre where they would learn there was no statistical or causal association between the two. There is a lesson here about the nature of medical facts, and our willingness to disregard the obvious until it is demonstrated in a large epidemiological study.

In the field of violence and mental health, the relevant epidemiology was Swanson et al.'s (1990) paper based on the Epidemiologic Catchment Area community sample of 10 000 people. Over a 12-month period violence was reported by 2% of those with no psychiatric diagnosis, by 8% of people with 'pure' schizophrenia, and by 13% whose schizophrenia was complicated by substance misuse or personality disorder. There is now a vast literature on violence and mental disorder (see Taylor, 1993 for an early summary) but Swanson's study used a representative sample and was of a high methodological standard.

The positive aspects of this study include the use of a large, community sample and accurate diagnosis. One weakness is the reliance on self-report, although subsequent work suggests that self-report is reasonably accurate. The McArthur study of mental disorder and violence, for example, went to considerable trouble to supplement self-report using records and informants, but unearthed very few additional incidents.

The findings need careful interpretation. They do not mean that schizophrenia (or alcoholism or personality disorder, for that matter) causes violence. The findings do show that patients with schizophrenia are at increased risk of behaving violently, compared with people with no psychiatric diagnosis. The increase in risk is not great, but it is statistically significant.

From that point on, the management of violence risk became a problem for mental health services. It is common for medical services to manage the complications of diseases. For example, one aim of treating diabetes is to minimize vascular, ocular, and other complications, and the proper management of hypertension is directed at reducing the occurrence of strokes. Psychiatry is just unfortunate that one complication of schizophrenia affects others as much as, or more than, it affects the patient. In other respects, management of a disease's complications is mainstream medical practice.

## Public expectations and attitudes

At the same time as psychiatry has been coming to terms with the fact that some mental disorders carry an increased risk of violence to others, all professionals have been the subject of increased scrutiny of their power and accountability. The assault on the power and privileges of doctors began with Foucault (1967) and Illich (1976) but has now moved out of sociology departments to become a strong theme in mainstream politics.

Consumerist attitudes to medicine have been strengthened by scandals such as that surrounding heart surgery for children in Bristol, UK (Bristol Royal Infirmary Inquiry, 2001), organ retention at Alder Hey, and the murder of patients by Harold Shipman. In Bristol, heart surgery for children had unacceptably high death rates, and these problems and concerns about the competence of the surgeon concerned were concealed from service users. At Alder Hey, organs removed from children at post mortem were retained without any consent, ostensibly in the name of research but apparently at the whim of the pathologist concerned. The Shipman case involved a GP who was able to kill patients repeatedly because of a lack of scrutiny and reluctance by other doctors to question suspicious behaviour.

While none of these cases involves psychiatry directly, doctors working in mental health had to respond to a changed climate in which the public no longer trusted doctors to take decisions about risk on their behalf. Alongside the dramatic, headline cases mentioned above has been a steady rise in concern about perceived racism and other discrimination within services. As implicit trust was lost, the emphasis shifted to informed consent, consultation, and transparency.

Psychiatry was in a weaker position to begin with as it never enjoyed the glamour attaching to surgeons and physicians, and it suffered from the stigmatization of the mentally ill. An added problem was that psychiatry grew up without the safety culture that was necessary in acute specialties of medicine and surgery. As something of a backwater, and as the career choice of more thoughtful and philosophical medical students, it was ill-prepared for external scrutiny of its management of violence risk.

The focus for these pressures on psychiatry since the early 1990s has been the independent Homicide Inquiry (see Chapter 3 for a detailed discussion). These Inquiries vary in quality but one of the themes running through many of them was the need for better assessment of violence risk.

Opinions vary on the value of homicide Inquiries and many clinicians loathe them. Nevertheless, in highlighting the need for a more systematic and transparent assessment of violence risk they are articulating a powerful political force. Any professional body that attempts to stand against that tidal wave, equipped with only an argument that amounts to: 'Trust me, I'm a doctor', can expect to be swept aside.

## There is no alternative ...

When popular politics joins with the financial might of the insurance companies, most professional resistance is bound to fall away. As corporate bodies, hospitals have had to adapt to a world in which errors or shortcomings lead to a lawsuit, with dire financial consequences even if it is successfully defended. Risk management has therefore become an important corporate activity. The practical consequence for mental health services has been that they have had violence risk management imposed upon them from above, often by people who know little about mental health or violence.

In most cases, the risk assessment amounts to a checklist on which boxes are ticked. There are often no instructions on how to complete it, or on what to do when it has been completed. When training is provided, many staff do not attend. This approach to violence risk assessment may be better than nothing, but it is not much better. It may give a false sense of security, and it is not a proper assessment of violence risk. The question posed for thinking clinicians is: If you have to do violence risk assessment (and you do), then why not do it properly?

## Summary: why worry about the assessment of violence risk

The objections to the assessment of violence risk include an ethical view that it is outside the proper limits of a doctor's role, or that mental capacity is a better alternative. In fact, many aspects of medical practice involve obligations and duties beyond any simple, exclusive relationship between doctor and patient, and the management of risk to third parties has precedents in other fields of medicine. Capacity cannot be separated from questions of risk and does not offer a true alternative.

Violence risk assessment is comparable with other risk assessments in medicine, and all are better than nothing. Quite apart from considerations of accuracy, structured risk assessment has the advantage of transparency and sits well with increasing pressure on professionals to open up their practice to external scrutiny.

Legal and commercial pressures, as well as public opinion, demand better risk assessments and the most persuasive argument in its favour may be that it is inevitable. Once that fact is accepted, the crucial questions concern the extent to which it can be improved, and the next chapter deals with research on the topic.

# Chapter 2

# Researching violence risk

Always protect your back
*The first law of forensic psychiatry (Anon.)*

## Violence and mental disorder

Research in this area is expanding rapidly. In fact, at the risk of provoking the response that some people are never satisfied, I would argue that until recently there was not enough research on the epidemiology of violence and mental disorder but now there is too much. I justify this statement by referring to the two basic rules of good epidemiology. First, ask a sensible and interesting question to which you do not already know the answer. Second, choose a sample that can answer it. Some recent research fails one or both of these tests.

An early and influential study compared rates of mental disorder in prisoners held on remand for violent and non-violent offences (Taylor and Gunn, 1984). Psychosis was much commoner in the violent group than could be explained by chance. These findings were in accord with clinical impressions in suggesting a link between psychosis and violence. The precise link in this study was with serious violence as many of the men in the sample were charged with offences at the upper end of the spectrum.

The limitation of the Taylor and Gunn study is its use of prisoners. It is not too great a limitation because most serious violence is likely to result in a remand to prison. Still, the ideal would have been a community sample if one could find the resources to make it large enough to include sufficient violent acts for statistical analysis. (In fact, over 20 years later, Shaw *et al.* (2006) did the equivalent of a community study to show that schizophrenia has a prevalence of 5% in homicide perpetrators in England and Wales, compared with 1% in the general population. This study was part of the National Confidential Inquiry into Suicides and Homicides and is discussed further in Chapter 3.)

The next major development was a community study by Swanson *et al.* (1990), who asked a sensible question and chose a perfect sample. In order to find out whether there was a statistical association between violence and various mental disorders, his team used the Epidemiologic Catchment Area (ECA) sample of about 10 000 people. The sample was drawn from and representative of the community, and it was large enough to give a reasonably accurate estimate of uncommon conditions and events. Psychiatric diagnoses were made as part of the larger ECA study and the rest of the methodology was simple. Researchers asked people if they had carried out any violent actions over the last 12 months. They found that violence was reported by 2% of those with no psychiatric diagnosis, by 8% of people with 'pure' schizophrenia, and by 13% whose schizophrenia was complicated by substance misuse or personality disorder.

There is now a vast literature on violence and mental disorder (see Taylor, 1993, for an early summary, and there has been much more since then) but Swanson's study remains a landmark. It changed orthodox teaching in mental health, and we continue to struggle with its consequences. The results showed that patients with schizophrenia were at an increased risk of behaving violently. Unless this was a coincidence, it meant that violence and violence risk assessment had to take a central place in mental healthcare.

It was inevitable and desirable that similar studies would follow, to see if the findings applied to other populations. In Sweden, Lindqvist and Allebeck (1990a,b) followed up 650 patients with schizophrenia and confirmed the association of schizophrenia with violence, as well as showing how much that risk was increased by drugs or alcohol.

In New York, Link et al. (1992) compared rates of arrest and self-reported violence in various groups of patients, with rates in a control group of people who had never had mental health treatment. The patient groups all had higher rates of violence, even after controlling for demographic factors.

In Israel, Stueve and Link (1997) found that a psychotic disorder of any type carried a relative risk of 3.3% for fighting and 6.6% for weapon use, after controlling for demographic factors, substance misuse, and antisocial personality disorder.

Studies of birth cohorts added to the weight of evidence. In Sweden, Hodgins (1992) found a fourfold increase in lifetime violent offences in those with a major mental disorder compared to those without. A Danish birth cohort (Hodgins et al. 1996; Brennan et al., 2000) consisting of all persons born between 1944 and 1947 (nearly 400 000 people) revealed a similar association between schizophrenia and violence. Arsenault et al. (2000) came up with similar findings in a birth cohort of 961 New Zealanders studied at the age of 21 years. Schizophrenia emerged with an odds ratio of 5.4 for violence (defined by self-report and/or convictions).

The alert reader will have noticed a repetitive quality creeping in to these findings and it is unnecessary to quote further studies. Faced with mounting evidence in the early 1990s, Monahan (1992) revised his earlier view and concluded that mental disorder was a significant and robust risk factor for community violence. Many of the studies since have done no more—but also no less—than confirm the original findings of Swanson *et al.*

By the mid-1990s, this line of research was no longer answering interesting questions. Its continued survival owed more to the research industry's need to generate product than to the pursuit of knowledge. Certainly clinicians who stopped paying attention in 1992 would not have missed anything important in this area. It is unlikely that hospital chief executives delayed the introduction of their violence risk management policy to await the outcome of the latest cohort study from Tunbridge Wells, Des Moines, or wherever.

In scientific terms, the existence of a link between mental disorder and violence is no longer controversial. In summary, there is a highly significant association between psychotic mental illness and violence in the community, of a similar order of magnitude to the association between smoking and lung cancer (Maden, 2004). There is an even stronger association of violence with psychopathy or antisocial personality disorder, and with drug or alcohol misuse. There is little point in reiterating these facts. The priority for research must be to find out more about how violence is linked to mental disorder, and what can be done to reduce violence in treatment populations.

## Research on violence risk prediction

The previous section dealt with the growing literature on violence and mental disorder. The next step is to examine the response of mental health professionals to the risk of violence. Violence risk is increased in some mental disorders, but the implications for clinical practice depend on whether we can estimate that risk with any accuracy. So how good are we at predicting violence? Do we know enough to start protecting ourselves from criticism? More importantly, do we know enough to be able to offer the public any of the protection that they, and their politicians, see as such an important part of the work of mental health services? Are we up to the job?

This is an important and not unreasonable question, but the research evidence is limited. At first glance it is not clear why this should be. After all, risk is a statistical concept that lends itself readily to large-scale outcome studies. There are, however, several reasons why we have few studies and many reservations about their findings.

The first problem is that serious violence is relatively rare, so any study has to be large and expensive in order to have any hope of picking up useful information. Large studies are good for detecting general causal factors and principles, but they are less good for looking at the details of clinical practice.

The second problem is that dispassionate scientific study is impossible given the need to prevent violence. If we predict serious violence we cannot sit and wait for it to happen. For the same reason, any discharge study faces the problem that a high violence risk tends to prevent discharge. It is no accident that some of the main studies in this area are naturalistic experiments, caused by events beyond the investigator's control (e.g. the Baxstrom case, discussed below). Inevitably, these circumstances lead to methodological limitations.

A third problem is that the research has often not been linked to clinical practice. Some of the landmark studies (e.g. Lidz *et al.*, 1993) are brilliant social science but seem to have adopted a policy of ignoring real-world clinical practice.

The final problem is that, until recently, neither clinicians nor researchers appeared interested in the question of violence risk prediction. Given the current prominence of the issue of violence, there are embarrassingly few studies that beleaguered clinicians can use to defend themselves against the charge of complacency.

An inevitable consequence of the dearth of relevant studies is that many people will already be familiar with those described in this section. In an attempt to avoid a simple rehash of old material, I try to show the relevance of these studies to modern practice. From that point of view, the things these studies do not tell us are as important as their findings. Researchers in this area often fail to address the questions that are important to clinicians.

## The link between mental illness and violence

An interesting and horrifying aspect of some violence by the mentally ill is its association with psychotic symptoms. To use some actual examples, a patient with no previous violence developed the delusion that his mother was the devil, so he killed her in order to save the world. A patient living a in a hostel interpreted sensations in his anus as definite evidence that his friend had sexually abused him during the night, so he confronted and killed him. A patient was convinced that a pending solar eclipse meant the end of the world, when people would turn on each other, so he stabbed several people in the street before they had the chance to attack him. Voices tell a man to attack, so he obeys them.

The point is that the symptoms appear to be the only motive for extreme violence. Some cases are more complicated, with mixed motives and origins in real disputes, but the purity of the pathological motivation in these cases is striking. We often speak of senseless or meaningless violence but here it is in archetypal form. This is violence flowing directly from an imbalance of brain chemicals, or faulty wiring in the brain, or a mixture of the two.

One of the central themes of this book is that not all violence is equal, and it is possible to attach values to different types of violence. I would argue that this type of violence, with clear psychotic motivation, is most important to mental health services, mainly because a good dose of antipsychotic medication goes a long way towards preventing it. Treatment has a dramatic, positive effect on outcome but, by the same token, a failure to treat can be disastrous.

## Delusions and violence

The link between psychotic symptoms and violence has stimulated a lot of research in recent years, although few revelations have emerged. Delusions, or fixed, false beliefs not explained by the individual's religious or cultural background, are an obvious target for such research. Hafner and Boker's (1982) large epidemiological survey in Germany found that delusions were associated with serious violence. Humphreys *et al.* (1992) reported on a cohort of patients whose schizophrenia presented with a serious violent act and found that in about 40% of cases the violence was motivated by delusions. Taylor *et al.'s* (1994) review found few relevant studies with plenty of methodological problems, including difficulty in measuring delusions.

Sampling is a problem in this field. If the study sample includes many non-psychotic patients who are violent, the apparent importance of delusions is reduced. One suspects this may have been an issue in Teplin *et al.'s* (1994) follow-up study of over 700 jail detainees, in whom delusions did not appear to be related to serious violent offending. One would expect a high level of violence in jail detainees, most of whom are not mentally ill, so it may not be the best place to look for the effects of delusions. A case control study, using relatively small numbers of violent vs. non-violent patients with schizophrenia, found the presence of delusions to be associated with violence (Cheung *et al.*, 1997).

Some research in this area has rather lost its way and failed one of the tests posed at the start of the chapter, by not using the correct sample for the question. If one wants to know about the importance of delusions as a risk factor for violence, the initial starting point should be a sample of patients with schizophrenia or another psychosis. Once you include patients without a psychotic disorder, the picture is obscured. The more non-psychotic, violent people you include, the less likely you are to find that delusions are associated with violence. The authors of the MacArthur study made this mistake when they went beyond the limits of what their sample could do and suggested delusions were not linked to violence. (Appelbaum *et al.*, 2000, discussed in more detail below.)

The only justification for a mixed sample of various diagnoses would be if one wanted to know how important delusions are as a cause of violence in the entire community, when the sample would have to be representative of the community. But we know the answer to that question—they are not very important in numerical terms—so there is little point in wasting time and money on it. Our main interest is in delusions in people with mental illness, and the extent to which those delusions are associated with violence. Here, the weight of evidence is strongly in favour of an association. I would refer to the clinical examples at the start of this section and challenge critics to show that delusions were not important in these cases. If they do not convince, the appropriate next step should be to compare violence rates by the same schizophrenic patients when they have delusions, with rates of violence when they do not have delusions. Delusions are, after all, a state rather than a trait variable, and use of patients as their own controls gets round all the matching problems. Nobody has done such a study, probably because we can all guess the results. We are right to assume that delusions are important in violence by the mentally ill, and we should move on to the more important question of what distinguishes those who act violently on the basis of their delusions, from those who do not.

Kendler *et al.* (1983) suggested that distress associated with delusions may help to explain increased violence risk, which is consistent with suggestions that associated anxiety (Buchanan, 1997) or anger are important (Appelbaum *et al.*, 2000). Buchanan *et al.* (1993) found that patients who acted on persecutory delusions in any way, not necessarily in a violent manner, tended to differ from those who did not act in that they could identify evidence in support of their delusion, they had actively searched for such evidence, and they were emotionally affected by their delusions. The associated emotion is important to clinicians. There is an element of tautology in the active search for supporting evidence, as it is another form of acting on the delusions, but it is an important practical way for clinicians to check for a sign of acting out that may not be obvious in observed behaviour. A review of the relationship between delusional misidentification and homicide suggested that the associated level of fear or anger is an indicator of risk (Silva *et al.*, 1995).

There are more papers in a similar vein but the point has been made. Delusional patients who are angry and upset about their beliefs, and who go looking for evidence, are more dangerous than those who are unperturbed by them and quietly get on with their lives. I suspect the same applies to political or religious beliefs, but it is still a useful observation if your job is to manage deluded people.

## Threat and control override

Another aspect of delusions that has become a focus for research is that of threat and control override (TCO). Link and Stueve (1994) used this term to refer to delusions that cause feelings of personal threat, and pathological thoughts that override self-control. The typical scenario is the persecutory delusion in which the sense of threat is used to justify pre-emptive action and overrides a person's normal inhibitions against violence. Hence the examples at the beginning of this section of the man killing his mother to save the world because the devil was in her, or the man attacking strangers out of a conviction that they were about to attack him.

Link *et al.* (1998, 1999) tested this hypothesis in retrospective case–control studies and found that other psychotic symptoms were unrelated to violence once they controlled for TCO symptoms. The 1998 paper also suggested that threat and control override symptoms were independent indicators of increased violence risk, which raises the question of why they remain linked in the TCO term. Swanson *et al.* (1996) compared violence in schizophrenics with and without TCO symptoms, and found rates of violence of 16% and 6%, respectively, a difference that is statistically significant.

This strand of research on delusions has yielded important and consistent findings with implications for clinical practice (I deal below with the apparent dissenting results in Appelbaum *et al.*, 2000).

## Developmental and personality factors

Many actuarial or structured clinical assessments of risk use indicators that relate to early development and to personality. Childhood developmental problems, disadvantage and abuse are associated with a propensity to violence in adulthood, irrespective of whether the person is mentally ill. Violence in schizophrenia is associated with educational problems and poor peer relationships in childhood and adolescence (Tihonen *et al.*, 1997; Fresan *et al.*, 2004). Conduct disorder in childhood has a strong association with schizophrenia, so much so that it is predictive of development of the disease (Gosden *et al.*, 2005). Schizophrenics with a history of conduct disorder are more likely to be violent than those without such a history.

Psychopathy is associated with increased violence risk, and for that reason features in many violence risk assessments. Its measurement in schizophrenia by means of the Hare Psychopathy Checklist (Hare, 1991) raises conceptual issues as some features of chronic schizophrenia mimic the lack of empathy and impulsivity that are characteristic of psychopathy.

There is other evidence to show that premorbid personality is associated with violence and other criminality in schizophrenia (e.g. Moran *et al.* 2003; Moran and Hodgins 2004). The picture is further complicated if it is acknowledged that schizophrenia may itself be a developmental disorder. Is the personality disorder seen before onset of the disease a separate entity or part of a single disease process? Fortunately, such complicated questions are beyond the scope of this paper. For our purposes, it is very convenient that several developmental and personality features act as markers for increased violence risk in schizophrenia, and are in some ways more useful in that regard than the symptoms considered above. These factors feature in later chapters on structured violence risk assessment. For now, it is appropriate to move on to a consideration of how well clinicians are able to assess the risk of violence.

## Can clinicians predict violence?

His story may be familiar to the point of cliché but any attempt to answer this question has to begin with Johnnie Baxstrom (Steadman and Keveles, 1972; Steadman and Cocozza, 1974). After a conviction for assault, Baxstrom was sent to prison in 1959 but later diagnosed as mentally ill and transferred to one of New York State's hospitals for the criminally insane. When his sentence expired in 1961 he was disappointed to learn that, instead of being released, he was to remain in hospital because he was still considered to be both mentally ill and dangerous. He petitioned the Supreme Court and in February 1966 the Court ordered his release.

Although the 5 years that elapsed between the end of his sentence and his release suggest the Court spent a long time pondering its decision, the lawyers were not considering the technicalities of risk assessment. The Court's decision was based entirely on Baxstrom's constitutional rights. Under the 14th Amendment, states are compelled to give their residents equal protection under the law and Baxstrom had been denied that protection as a result of his mental illness.

Baxstrom's personal triumph became of wider interest when New York State realized that 966 other detained patients in their hospitals for the criminally insane could petition the Supreme Court on the same grounds and could expect to win. They gave in gracefully and ordered that all 967 patients should be transferred to civil mental hospitals within the space of a few months.

Good law made for great science. These patients, who could have expected to be detained for years because of a perceived high risk of violence, were released from secure hospitals for purely legal reasons. No ethical committee would contemplate approving a scientific study of this type, so researchers rushed to take advantage of the natural experiment.

Steadman and various colleagues (1972, 1974) followed up the Baxstrom patients for 4 years and found only 16 convictions in total, involving nine patients out of a sample, for these purposes, of 246. Only two of the 16 convictions were for felonies, namely one assault and one robbery. At the end of the follow-up period about half of the patients were still in civil mental hospitals, 27% had been discharged to the community and 14% were dead. Only 3% of the original group were back in prisons or forensic hospitals, although 20% were violent on at least one occasion during the follow-up.

Even without further information, several points can be made. First, the hospitals for the criminally insane appear to have been over-cautious when recommending further detention. The risks presented by this group of patients over a 4-year period were manageable without recourse to such a high level of security. In fact, despite the high level of public anxiety about violence by patients, mental health services are generally very cautious about discharging patients who have been labelled as dangerous. The rate of serious offending in conditionally discharged restricted patients in England and Wales is about 0.6% per annum (Home Office, 2001).

The second point to make is that these patients were not all safe to be in the community. Half remained in hospital throughout the 4-year follow-up, which probably contributed to the low rate of serious violence. Despite the low level of convictions, one in five patients were violent. This is a high proportion and serves as a reminder that violence in the context of mental disorder may be difficult to study because much of it is never processed through the courts.

Could psychiatrists have predicted which of the patients would fall into the violent group? Steadman and Cocozza (1974) found that six characteristics tended to predict violence (Table 2.1).

Cocozza and Steadman (1976) used these findings to develop a Legal Dangerousness Scale, which they applied to all patients released into the community. High scores were obtained for most patients who later behaved violently but, for every violent patient, two others had similar scores but did not

**Table 2.1** Predictors of violence during four-year follow-up of the Baxstrom patients (Steadman and Cocozza, 1974)

| |
| --- |
| History of juvenile offending |
| Number of previous arrests |
| Previous convictions |
| Previous convictions for violence |
| Severity of the original offence |
| Age (–) |

behave violently. In other words, for every true positive there were two false positives.

The authors make the point that in order to minimize the total error rate the best statistical strategy is to predict that none of the group will be violent. This ensures there will be no false positives and, because violence is relatively rare, the false negative rate will be low. Any other strategy will pick up some true positives but this gain will be outweighed by a greater increase in false positives.

Modern mental health services, looking after populations with low rates of serious violence, face this inescapable dilemma. The statistics dictate that any attempt to predict violence will lead to more errors than hits. Some people argue from this observation that we should abandon any attempt to predict violence, but that despairing position is untenable because mental health services deal with people rather than abstract mathematical events. As Monahan (1981) has pointed out, statistical reasoning assumes that all errors are of equal importance. The task of clinicians is to assign costs, weights, and values to different types of error. The consequences of being overcautious in prolonging the detention of a patient are quite different from the consequences of discharging a patient who goes on to kill. Like it or not, we have to estimate the risk of violence as best we can.

Turning to the question of how well we can estimate the risk of violence, much of the early research on risk prediction offers little comfort. Another famous study is an international survey in which psychiatrists and other professionals were asked to rate 16 case histories for dangerousness (Harding and Montandon, 1982, Montandon and Harding, 1984). Agreement between the 193 raters ranged from 35% to 86% but the 62 psychiatrists did not agree among themselves any more than did other professionals.

Of course, this was not a study of whether the predictions were accurate. In scientific terms, it was concerned with reliability (do different raters agree?) rather than validity (are they right?). The reasoning behind the study, quite correctly, is that there is no point in even asking whether psychiatrists get it right if members of the profession cannot get as far as agreeing on an answer.

One could spend a lot of time listing the limitations of this study. It used case histories, which are not the only basis of risk assessments in real life. An international sample was likely to increase disagreement, given differences in service organization, training, and experience. But such nitpicking obscures the important point. The findings of this study are consistent with information from other sources, and we have to accept that unstructured, clinical judgement is an unreliable way to assess violence risk.

For me, the surprising thing about the Harding and Montandon study is that there was such good agreement, as most participants had probably had no specific training in the assessment of dangerousness. Perhaps we are better at this business than we think we are. My other comment is that this paper belongs to an earlier age, when the assessment of dangerousness was a specialist, esoteric activity of little everyday relevance. It shows a proper sense of concern about the limits to medical expertise but there is no sense of urgency, and there is no consideration of the implications for services of psychiatrists being unable to agree. This study has been presented as an argument for throwing in the towel when faced with problems of risk assessment, whereas a service manager would respond by asking how to train staff to reach a better level of agreement.

As risk assessment is now a central concern for services, studies in the real world are bound to be of more interest. One of the best early examples was carried out in a psychiatric emergency room in the USA. Lidz *et al.* (1993) looked at 357 patients in whom emergency room psychiatrists predicted violence, along with 357 matched controls, in whom the same psychiatrists did not predict violence. Over a 6-month follow-up period, violence was measured by self-report and by collateral reports. Violence occurred in 53% of the predicted cases and in 36% of the control group.

This study is important first for showing that violence was more common than many other studies had suggested, occurring in 45% of all cases. Even when allowance is made for the emergency room setting, this is a high proportion. Almost every other person seen by the psychiatrist went on to commit a violent act within a few months of the consultation, a statistic that ought to concentrate the mind of anyone regularly carrying out assessments of this type.

The study also showed that the predictions were considerably better than chance, with violence occurring in just over half the cases in which it had been predicted. Clinicians did less well with patients in whom they did not predict violence as just over a third of them did, in fact, go on to commit a violent act. To put these results into statistical terms, the false positive rate was just under one in two, but the false negative rate was just over one in three.

This is an excellent and influential study and definitely passes the tests for good question and right sample. Its strengths include the large sample, use of controls from the same population, and a naturalistic setting.

On the other hand, it has one massive limitation, in that it says nothing about treatment or its effect on outcome. This is particularly surprising to clinicians in the UK, where practice is increasingly dominated by concern about violence. As the possibility of violence is one of the main indications for psychiatric intervention, there would usually be at least an offer of treatment if violence appeared likely at an emergency assessment. As litigation against doctors is virtually a sport in the USA, it is inconceivable that there would be no thought given to intervention when violence was predicted.

If one assumes that there must have been treatment intervention in at least some of the cases, then the results are open to different interpretations. Did the 'predicted violence' group get more treatment and the control group less? If so, would the rates of violence have been even higher without intervention? Would the difference between the groups have been greater, if there had been no intervention whatever the perceived risk of violence?

One can only speculate on these matters. What is certain is that researchers who conducted an otherwise excellent study did not include any mention of intervention, which clinicians may well see as the most important of all possible influences on violence. This problem runs throughout the literature in this field. The Lidz study was a success in its own terms and it answered the questions it posed, so one should not be too critical of the authors for not choosing to do a different study. However, there are grounds for criticism of the research community in general, for failing to give sufficient attention to the impact of psychiatric services. It is more than 10 years since the Lidz paper was published, but there is still very little in the literature about the impact of treatment on violence risk (Steadman, 2000).

## The MacArthur violence risk assessment study

The MacArthur study is the largest study to examine risk factors for violence in patients in the community. It consists of a descriptive, 12-month follow-up of 1136 men and women discharged from general psychiatric hospitals in three US cities, and it cost about $8 million. This amounts to almost $8000 per patient, and a large part of these considerable resources went into efforts to measure violence accurately, and to collect as much data as possible on factors likely to relate to violence risk. The authors measured 134 separate variables in order to determine their links and interactions in relation to the main outcome measure, which was violence.

Semi-structured interviews before discharge were followed by interviews in the community every 10 weeks. Primary research diagnoses at baseline are shown in Table 2.2. I include this information because, to paraphrase the estate agents' motto, the three most important features of any epidemiological study are the sample, the sample, and the sample. I will make repeated reference to the sample because it accounts for the strengths and the flaws of this study, and it is impossible to make sense of the findings without taking account of the particular features of the study population.

The researchers used several standardized instruments, some of which were developed for the study. The most important of these specially developed measures is probably the PCL-SV or Psychopathy Checklist—Screening Version (Hart et al., 1995). It was expected that personality disorder, and

**Table 2.2** Baseline research diagnoses in the MacArthur Violence Risk Assessment Study (%, *n* = 1136)

| | |
|---|---|
| Depression/dysthymia | 40.3 |
| Alcohol or drug abuse/dependence | 23.9 |
| Schizophrenia/schizoaffective disorder | 17.2 |
| Bipolar disorder | 13.3 |
| Other psychiatric disorder | 3.5 |
| Personality disorder only | 1.8 |

psychopathy in particular, would be strongly associated with violence, so there was a need for a reliable and valid measure of psychopathy that was suitable for use in a non-forensic population and was quicker to administer than the full PCL-R. There is further discussion of psychopathy and these checklists in Chapter 5.

One purpose of the patient interviews was to obtain a detailed self-report of violent behaviour, which was also measured using informants (relatives or key workers) and official records. These extra sources of information increased the detection of violence but self-report was reasonably effective on its own, and revealed a lot of violence that was never documented in official records. This is good news for clinicians or, at least, good news for clinicians who ask their patients about violent behaviour.

The analysis of this mass of data had two purposes. The first aim was to describe violence in this group of patients and to identify those factors that were associated with the violence and may therefore help in predicting it. The second major aim was to develop a standardized risk assessment instrument, in the form of a decision tree (described by the authors as an Iterative Classification Tree) that assigns patients to a high- or low-risk group. As this is an attempt at actuarial or standardized risk assessment, it will be considered in Chapter 5.

## The main findings of MacArthur

Even from this brief account, it is obvious that the MacArthur study is an impressive undertaking, and it would be easy to be seduced into thinking of it as the last word on violence and mental disorder. So what does it tell us about violence by psychiatric patients?

### Violence is common in mental health populations

Assaults were common in this group of patients, committed by nearly 30% over the year. That percentage lies in the same range as the Lidz emergency room sample (see above). As with the Lidz study, one's first response is surprise; that is a lot of violence. Still, some qualification is necessary.

Managed care meant that most admissions were brief, with patients still suffering symptoms of the index episode at the point of discharge. Much of the violence was probably associated with the initial, acute episode. The number of patients committing violence decreased rapidly in the early phase of the study, falling from 13.5% at the first follow-up to 6.9% by the third. About 30% of the sample had probable or definite delusions at baseline, although this figure had fallen to about 17% at the first follow-up and only 12% had delusions by the end of the study.

Perhaps more importantly, less than 10% of all the violent acts occurred when a patient was psychotic. Most violence occurred at home and the victims were usually family or friends.

## Substance misuse is more important then mental illness as a cause of violence

The second striking finding was that once substance misuse was excluded, patients did not have increased rates of violence compared with other people in their community. Substance misuse increased rates of violence in both patient and non-patient groups. However, substance misuse was commoner in the patient group so, unless the analysis allows for that fact, it is easy to get the impression that violence is commoner among patients *per se* (Steadman *et al.*, 1998).

This finding has been misinterpreted, not least by the authors themselves, to suggest that mental illness is not associated with violence once substance abuse is taken out of the picture. This is true for the sample concerned, in which almost a quarter of the patients have a primary diagnosis of substance misuse, but it is not true as a general statement. As there is so much substance misuse in the sample, once it is taken out of the picture little remains from which to draw any meaningful conclusions. We know already, from numerous studies with larger and more appropriate samples (e.g. Swanson *et al.*, 1990), that mental illness is important in its own right as a causal factor in violence. Incidentally, the Swanson study also made the point that substance abuse was generally more important than mental illness as a cause of violence.

## Psychopathy is a useful predictor of violence in general mental health populations

The third major finding was that psychopathy, as measured by the PCL-SV, was the best single predictor of violence. The success of the PCL-SV as a predictor of violence in a non-forensic population could be considered the most important finding of the entire project. Most research on the predictive value of the Psychopathy Checklist had been done in prison or forensic psychiatric populations, which have higher rates of psychopathy. That research shows that a diagnosis of psychopathy is associated with increased risk of recidivism or offending in general, and of violence in particular. In the MacArthur study very few patients had scores high enough to qualify for the label of psychopathy, yet their psychopathy scores still had discriminatory power in relation to violence risk. The psychopathy trait therefore has important predictive value, even in a normal population. The implication of this finding is that the measurement of psychopathy is important not only to forensic psychiatrists who work with offender populations, but to general psychiatrists as well.

Given the importance of substance misuse, it may seem surprising that psychopathy comes out as the best single predictor. Of course there is enormous overlap, with a higher prevalence of substance misuse correlating with higher psychopathy scores.

In any case, it is pointless to become preoccupied by the search for the Holy Grail of the 'best' predictor. The value of these factors for the clinician is in their coexistence and interaction. For example, if you work with a population of substance abusers, that characteristic alone is of little value in assessing relative risk. It may be more helpful to know their psychopathy scores. When assessing risk in substance misusers with high psychopathy scores, variables such as mental state and anger become important as discriminatory variables.

## Violence in mental health populations is related to many of the same factors as in the general population

The fourth important finding of the MacArthur study was that, in addition to psychopathy and the misuse of substances, violence was linked to previous violence, to neighbourhood context, and to anger, as well as to the usual demographic variables of age and sex. These findings are consistent with the general literature on violence and they are not specific to violence associated with mental disorder. Given the low prevalence of assaults directly associated with psychosis, one could summarize the results of this study as showing that the violent behaviour of psychiatric patients is, for most of the time, pretty much the same as the violent behaviour of their non-patient neighbours. Most violence by discharged patients has the same motivations as other violence in that community, and can be understood according to the same rules. This is, in itself, an important finding with far-reaching implications. At the same time, it reminds us of the limits to the study.

## Limitations of the MacArthur study

Before considering details, it is useful to start with value judgements. What do we want to achieve, and how do the findings of this study help? I have already quoted Monahan's reminder that not all errors are of equal value. If one extends this principle, it follows that not all violence is of equal importance to mental health services. We need to draw a line, and to be clear that mental health services are not society's main response to the problem of violence. They are not even a major part of that response, as mental disorder is a relatively unimportant cause of violence from a public health perspective.

### The wrong type of violence?

The starting point of this book is that mental health services have to be interested in violence because it is a preventable complication of some types of mental disorder. It follows that we are most interested in the violence that is closely associated with mental disorder. From that perspective, most of the assaults reported in the MacArthur study are the wrong type of violence. Of course, we need to be interested in all aspects of our patients' lives. We need to remember that violence risk is higher in angry young men from violent neighbourhoods, especially when they drink or take drugs, but we are essentially spectators in this particular show. Successful psychiatric rehabilitation amounts to returning a patient to the life he or she had before the onset of the mental illness, and in many cases that life has a lot of risk factors for violence. This is the world in which we practice, but it is not the target of our practice.

On the other hand, we need to know much more about the violence arising directly from mental illness and, in particular, from psychosis. Because this type of incident was relatively uncommon, the MacArthur study has only limited information to reveal.

### The right sample for the right question?

The MacArthur study is also not the place to look for basic knowledge about the association between violence and mental disorder. While MacArthur is often mentioned in the same context as Swanson *et al.* (1990) and the ECA study, they are based on entirely different samples. The ECA study was a representative community sample and can tell us more about the nature of mental disorder and violence. MacArthur used a sample of patients, a socially defined category not representative of all people with a particular disease or disorder.

To take one obvious example of possible bias by exclusion, MacArthur included no forensic patients. As it consisted of discharged patients, it has nothing to say about patients who were not discharged, or those who were not admitted in the first place. There is an arbitrary quality to the sample. If for example, the hospitals concerned had decided not to offer an inpatient service for patients whose primary diagnosis is drug or alcohol misuse/dependence—a defensible clinical decision—then the sample would have been quite different. None of this invalidates the results of the study, which is a brilliant description of a particular group of patients. However, it should make us think carefully before drawing general conclusions about the risk of violence in mental illness.

Which brings us to one area of the study where the findings are, as a result of these limitations, potentially misleading. The authors state, 'the presence of delusions does not predict higher rates of violence among recently discharged psychiatric patients' (Appelbaum *et al.*, 2000). That statement is true in their sample, but there are many reasons to doubt that it can be generalized to other settings. The study is not designed to answer questions about delusions, partly because of the case mix. The sample is heavily weighted for diagnoses in which delusions are most unlikely but violence is common. The more non-psychotic patients there are in a sample, the less likely it is to reveal any association between violence and delusions. And what about those psychotic patients who did not get into the sample because they were labelled as forensic cases? The presence of worrying delusions leads clinicians to assume that a patient is dangerous, thereby introducing systematic bias. If one wanted to answer questions about the importance of delusions as an indicator of risk in recently discharged patients, a better design would have been to follow a cohort of mentally ill patients to show how violence and delusions change over time.

I have devoted space to the dispute over delusions because the relationship between psychotic symptoms and violence is so important for mental health services. It is a question of values. The world may not judge us too harshly if our patients get into fights because they are drunk, but it is likely to take a dim view of any violence resulting from poor management of psychotic symptoms. This study provides little help to clinicians in understanding the role of delusions in violence by the mentally ill.

### And what about treatment?

The other disappointment for clinicians is the scant attention paid by MacArthur to treatment. The sample was defined by treatment status, as it consisted of recently discharged patients, so it is suitable for an inquiry into treatment rather than a general investigation of the characteristics of mental disorder. The study lets this opportunity pass and relies on self-reported experience of treatment, defined in broad terms as talking or medication. There is no information on the type of medication, or the type of talking treatment for that matter, and there is nothing on compliance or reasons for discontinuing treatment. These omissions are frustrating because the results suggest that treatment does make a difference; patients who received more of it were less likely to be violent in the following 10 weeks, at least in the early stages of the study.

## Conclusions

The MacArthur risk assessment study is a major work with excellent methodology. In many ways it represents the last word on this topic, in providing a detailed description of the factors associated with violence by psychiatric patients. Its findings are largely consistent with what we know from other sources, confirming gender, age, personality, previous violence, substance misuse and cultural influences as important determinants of violence. It is unreasonable to expect research to yield much more useful information on these topics.

On the other hand, clinicians can look at this body of work and feel disappointed, not to mention irritated. The unanswered questions are all about the details of clinical practice and, in particular, about intervention. The controversial 'findings' on mental illness, substance misuse, and violence, and on the relationship between delusions and violence, are methodological artefacts. They serve only to sow confusion in areas where frontline services need clear advice.

It is easy to criticize researchers for an apparent lack of interest in clinical issues, but there are real obstacles to research in this area. Even in a study as large and expensive as Macarthur, only 10% of violence occurred when patients were psychotic. This leaves the sample size looking rather less impressive. If we wanted to subdivide this sample, to start comparing different aspects of the psychotic state, or differences in management, we would need massive samples. The detailed documentation of treatment interventions would also be a major undertaking.

We come back to the methodological problem of the rarity of serious violence in mental illness. One of our major concerns in mental health services is to avoid an act of serious violence that leads to a homicide. We look to research to guide us but the MacArthur study included no homicides, and we cannot assume the factors associated with a psychotic killing will be the same as those associated with more mundane acts of less serious violence. The problem is not just that existing research has little to offer, but that we will also need to have modest expectations of future research because of the methodological difficulties.

As a possible way out of this dilemma, Chapter 3 looks at UK Homicide Inquiries as an additional source of information about violence by psychiatric patients. These Inquiries lack the scientific rigour of research and their methods are sometimes dubious, but they have the advantage of being firmly targeted at the details of clinical practice.

## Chapter 3

# When things go wrong ... Homicide Inquiries in the United Kingdom

## Introduction

In 1994 the UK Government responded to the publication of the Inquiry into the care and treatment of Christopher Clunis by issuing guidance making it mandatory for health services to hold an independent Inquiry into all cases of homicide by a patient who had been in recent contact with specialist mental health services (Department of Health, 1994). The reports were to be commissioned and paid for by the Health Authority responsible for the service concerned. Most Inquiry panels were chaired by a senior lawyer or judge and included a psychiatrist and a third person, usually with a background in social services or nursing. Some Inquiries had more members and others commissioned expert advice on particular aspects of a case. Most were held in private but some heard evidence in public.

The decision to hold such Inquiries was unpopular with psychiatrists from the start, and their opposition grew stronger as the reports multiplied. Media attention was inevitably most intense when Inquiries were critical of services or individuals. Some Inquiries revealed shocking failures, but there was plenty of room for argument about who was to blame. Were these the mistakes of individuals, or systemic failures in a Cinderella service whose meagre resources were devoted to priorities other than the prevention of violence?

The professions and the Government became polarized in a bitter debate about the effects of the policy. Was it a disaster that distorted priorities, damaged morale and made it harder to fill the many vacant posts in general psychiatry? Or did Inquiries draw attention to poor services and help to generate the massive increase in funding for mental health services over the last decade? It may be too soon to say whether the Inquiries have been good or bad for mental health services in the UK. The exponential growth of forensic mental health services over this period was probably no coincidence, but opinion within the profession is equally divided on the question of whether more forensic psychiatry is good or bad news.

Whatever the initial effects, a consensus grew that the Inquiry reports were becoming repetitive, with diminishing benefits to set against the costs and the negative publicity. The compromise solution was to establish in 1996 the National Confidential Inquiry into Suicide and Homicide by People with Mental Illness. The aim was to extend to mental health the methods used to investigate serious adverse outcome in other branches of medicine, such as maternal deaths in childhood. The mental health professions were grateful for the decreased attention given to individual services and staff. They also welcomed the linking of homicides and suicides, the latter being a far more common complication of mental illness. The Inquiry continues to gather data and to publish regular reports designed to improve practice in dealing with violence risk (Appleby *et al.*, 1999, 2001). The first two reports are discussed briefly at the end of this chapter.

The era of independent homicide Inquiries may be drawing to a close, but that is no reason to forget them. The purpose of this chapter is to extract from this vast literature some useful messages about the way we assess and manage risk. By contrast with much of the research literature, the homicide Inquiries can claim to mirror the reality of clinical practice, and it would be a serious mistake to ignore the picture they reflect back to us, however unpalatable it may be.

## What is wrong with independent Inquiries?

The debate on Inquiries has become polarized, with opponents tending to present them as an invention of the devil from which no good can ever come. The truth is that they have some good points and many bad ones, so before we consider what can be learned from them it is a good idea to set out the major problems.

1. **Reliance on the wisdom of hindsight.** It is easy to come along after the event and tell people what they should have done to avoid it. It is much more difficult to see things from the perspective of those who were doing the job at the time. Too many Inquiries constructed events to make a narrative in which the outcome was inevitable, then blamed those involved for not taking action earlier.

   Probably the worst offender in this respect was *The Falling Shadow* (Blom-Cooper *et al.*, 1995) a homicide Inquiry that the team decided to publish as a book. Even the title conveys a sense of predictability and inevitability that could not have been apparent to any of the people looking after the patient.

2. **Overemphasis on individual rather than systemic explanations.** Lawyers chair Inquiries, and lawyers are trained in establishing individual responsibility in criminal or civil trials. They are not trained to look at problems in terms of systems or resources. This is no bad thing, and we would be disappointed if a judge reached the end of a murder trial only to pronounce in his summing up that there is no point in pursuing individual responsibility because society is to blame. However, Inquiries into complex systems are different, and the individuals singled out for criticism will often look more like scapegoats than perpetrators.

Some Inquiries fail in two ways, by damaging morale through unfair criticism of individuals, and by failing to identify the underlying factors that need to be changed if similar incidents are to be avoided. The damage to morale goes beyond particular individuals, because others are affected by the knowledge that they could end up in the same position. This is the 'blame culture' identified by Szmukler (2000) and there is no doubting the damage that has been inflicted on services. Recognition of that damage has led the NHS to adopt Root Cause Analysis as the standard approach to reviews of critical incidents, in an attempt to go beyond the particular circumstances to identify underlying causes.

3. **Variable standards and poor quality control.** The trappings of the Inquiry process would have us believe their findings were found on tablets of stone at the top of a high mountain. However, the great advantage of science over law is that it defers to no expert authority. If clinicians are asked to take seriously the lessons of Inquiries, they can reasonably apply critical scrutiny to Inquiry reports just as they would to any other publication. Some reports stand up well to that process but some do not, because they are not very good. There are no established procedures for selecting members. As the Inquiry process is time-consuming, the medical member is often retired, and it is easy for a doctor to lose touch with the reality of clinical practice after leaving the fray. Forensic psychiatrists are sometimes asked to consider patients looked after by general psychiatrists, and vice versa. Neither general nor forensic psychiatrist is likely to have had specific training in how to do an Inquiry, so they tend to defer to the lawyer.

Inquiry chairmen have also varied in their interpretation of the role, with some being more ambitious than others. I have already mentioned the Falling Shadow Inquiry, which became a book (Blom-Cooper *et al.*, 1995). This Inquiry team took a wide view of its powers and duties. It devoted considerable energies to exploration of the law and the limits of the powers available to doctors in deciding when to intervene and detain a patient whose mental state is deteriorating.

A problem arises when these wider questions conflict with the investigation of the specific incident. It is unreasonable to expect the personnel concerned in an ordinary clinical decision to be operating at the cutting edge of legal practice, yet the Falling Shadow Inquiry's views were later challenged in a discussion paper from the Mental Health Act Commission (Eldergill, 1998). The point is not which view is correct, but that this esoteric debate belongs in legal journals and is out of place in an Inquiry that may blight the lives and careers of the individuals concerned. Similar tensions run through many Inquiries and raise questions about the extent to which their authors attempt to make general points at the expense of fairness in commenting on a particular incident.

4. **Cost.** Inquiries are expensive, and are bound to evoke envy in those who work in cash-strapped services.

Peay (1996) contains a fuller discussion of these problems. Munro (2004) welcomes a shift in the health service to an emphasis on systemic factors rather than individual actions as causes of error. She argues that homicide Inquiries should soften their emphasis on individual actions and would be more useful if they viewed human error as a symptom rather than a cause. The logical extension of this approach is to look at the systemic factors acting on the professional and consider whether they made a mistake more likely. This is a persuasive argument for Root Cause Analysis, although the two approaches need not be mutually exclusive.

Approaching the task of criticism from a new angle, Goldberg (2005) focused on one Inquiry and analysed it as a literary text. The events leading to the homicide were seen as a narrative constructed by the Inquiry, whereas the recommendations concerned bureaucratic change. An individual narrative may not be the best way to address the need for change in a complex bureaucracy.

It will be apparent by now that much of the published comment on Inquiries is negative. This is no surprise. Professional groups have a strong instinct for self-defence and rarely thank critics, irrespective of the merits of the criticism. However, in a world hostile to professional privilege, survival will depend on something more than a closing of the ranks. Mental health services need to put to one side their injured feelings and give more thought to some of the findings of the Inquiries. For all their faults, the best Inquiries are excellent case studies that tell us things about risk management we could not learn elsewhere. The following section summarizes the key findings of a few Inquiries, before considering a more systematic approach to learning from them.

## Homicides in perspective

Before considering homicides by psychiatric patients, it is helpful to remember the context. Taylor and Gunn (1999) carried out a trends analysis on criminal statistics for England and Wales between 1957 and 1995, to show that there was little fluctuation in the numbers of mentally ill people committing homicides over this period. As a result of a steady increase in other types of homicide, there was a 3% annual decline in their contribution to the overall statistics for homicide.

These findings, combined with the National Confidential Inquiry's demonstration that killings of strangers by the mentally ill are rare, should help to calm public fears about an epidemic of violence by the mentally ill. The overall violence risk attributable to mental illness is low, and a public health approach would undoubtedly give greater priority to the violence associated with, for example, alcohol or domestic disputes. On the other hand, low is not the same as insignificant. There is a unique horror about the killing of a stranger for psychotic motives. Such motives are perhaps the most pointless and incomprehensible of all reasons for a violent death. As some cases of schizophrenia present with an act of serious violence, and as some violent acts occur with no warning, it is inevitable that a small number of people will have to endure the grief that comes with knowing that a relative died in this way. Their suffering should never be compounded by the failure of mental health services to take seriously the risk of violence, or the failure to provide appropriate care when such a risk is identified. People who work in mental health services should be interested in violence by the mentally ill not because it is common, but because it concerns the efficacy of treatment and some of it is preventable.

## Examples of homicide Inquiries

The following have been chosen because they were landmarks in one way or another, or because they make a useful point. The first one, on the Clunis case, is here to illustrate the huge gulf between research and clinical practice in risk management. The previous chapter on research was concerned with the limits of our ability to assess and manage risk. Researchers attempted to tease out links between mental disorder and violence, grappling with complex statistics and models for understanding medical predictions and errors. Now, after the Lord Mayor's parade comes the little man with a shovel. The Ritchie report revealed the reality of risk management as reckless, high stakes gambling. This was Russian roulette with other people's lives, and you do not need Signal Detection Theory to understand the errors.

## The care and treatment of Christopher Clunis

Christopher Clunis killed Jonathan Zito on 17 December 1992. At about 4 p.m. on an ordinary Thursday afternoon, he stabbed the victim in the eye with no warning. His motivation was psychotic.

I have already referred to the case and the Inquiry several times, as it led to the Department of Health insisting that independent Inquiries should be mandatory after homicides by mental health patients. Although the case is notorious and frequently quoted, it justifies a more detailed treatment here for several reasons. First, some of the lessons of the Inquiry have still not permeated all of our mental health practice. Second, one of the themes of the report is that services made false assumptions about Christopher Clunis without bothering to check the facts. I suspect that many people who have not read the report still believe in the stereotypes. Third, it is a good report and a model of its kind. If I were asked what single document would most help a clinician to improve his or her management of violence risk, I would be inclined to recommend this one.

### Clunis's personal history

He was born in London in 1963 to Jamaican parents. He grew up within an intact and supportive family. He attended ordinary local schools and obtained several O levels before going on to Sixth Form College to study for A levels but he left before completing the course to pursue his long-held interest in a career in music, at which he had some success. He first showed symptoms of mental illness in 1986, when he turned 23, and he had his first admission to a hospital in Jamaica where he was diagnosed as suffering from schizophrenia. From the beginning he had poor self-care and violence occurred early in the illness: '... out of the blue, while the family were watching television together, he attempted to hit one of his nieces when she changed the programme' (Ritchie *et al.*, 1994, p. 9).

### Clunis's mental health care in London

As noted above, his first admission was in Jamaica. No details are available beyond the diagnosis. After that first admission, all his contact with services was in London.

- ◆ **1st contact.** In June 1987 his sister took him to the Emergency Dept of Chase Farm, a hospital in north London: '... he was in a terrible state, filthy, underweight, uncommunicative, confused, disorientated, staring into space, laughing and giggling to himself' (Ibid, p. 11). The duty psychiatrist made a diagnosis of schizophrenia, offered admission, and when it was refused arranged an emergency assessment at his sister's home by a Community Psychiatric Nurse (CPN) from the team serving that area.

- **2nd contact.** After further deterioration he had his first admission to Chase Farm from 2 to 27 July. During the admission he was suspected to have a drug-induced psychosis although a drug screen was negative. He was discharged after he was rude and over-familiar with female staff and patients. His sister thought (rightly) that he had been discharged too early. He was given no outpatient appointment and there were no arrangements for follow-up care. The housing department contacted the hospital in August and were informed the diagnosis was either mental illness or drug-induced psychosis (despite the negative drug screen).

- **2nd admission.** In December he presented in a deteriorated and dishevelled state, having been homeless for 2 weeks. He was discharged after 2 days with a diagnosis of a transient psychotic state because he appeared to have settled. There was no follow-up or contact with GP or family.

- **3rd contact.** In January the police brought him to hospital and he was admitted for 3 days, during which he assaulted two patients but seemed to respond to medication. The diagnosis was 'drug-induced? psychosis with no fixed abode'—and no evidence of drug use, I would add; no evidence of follow-up after discharge either.

- **4th contact.** In February he presented in a dishevelled state with a diagnosis of 'defect state schizophrenia' and was admitted for 4 days.

- **5th contact.** He was in prison in March 1988, when the prison wrote to the hospital for details of his treatment. No other information is available.

- **6th contact.** In March 1988 he went to the Emergency department because he was homeless. He was diagnosed as psychotic or schizoaffective illness but not thought to need acute admission. Attempts were made to provide social work help but they came to nothing.

- **Inquiry comment.** The Inquiry was critical of the fact that every contact was treated as if he were a new patient, with no attempt to reach a definitive diagnosis or to address his obvious needs.

- **7th Contact.** On 26 April 1988 he was arrested for stealing two loaves of bread and ended up miles from his home area in a bail hostel in south London. The probation officer took him to King's College Hospital immediately because he was 'talking to himself and laughing, refusing to eat or drink, making inappropriate contact with females and exposing himself'. He was diagnosed as psychotic and requiring admission, which finally came about on 3 May and he remained in hospital until 12 May. The doctor contacted Chase Farm but the doctor there said there was doubt about the diagnosis of schizophrenia and he was 'a difficult young man who just wanted a bed ... the hospital was unwilling to take responsibility for him because they did not regard him as psychotic'. He was discharged after several violent incidents on the ward with no accommodation but an outpatient appointment for July. He relapsed within 12 days of discharge, and on 25 May was arrested after breaking into the home of an elderly lady, where he was found in her bathroom. This was the last offence with which he was charged before his arrest for murder over 4 years later. It led to a hospital order but he was discharged within 16 days of admission while still unwell, with no proper aftercare.

I have given details up to this point because they convey the nature of his involvement with services. Clunis was not a patient who was lost to services for long periods of time. He could not cope in the community and he was always turning up at hospital or being brought by relations (in the early months) then police, probation or housing.

It would take a long time to recount the details of the subsequent 4 years of contact with services and they are detailed in the Inquiry report, which is an excellent summary. Table 3.1 lists some of the most striking points about his treatment.

The story of Clunis's mental health care is not an easy one to summarize, because there were so many failings over such a long period of time. By the time of the killing he had been in touch with services in London for $5^1/_2$ years, and most of his management was unsatisfactory. Most homicide Inquiries can be reduced to a few key issues. Should the depot have been stopped? Should the patient have been kept in hospital? Should there have been better follow-up? The Clunis case has hundreds of questions of this type, if you wanted to document them all. It is almost incredible that disaster did not come sooner, as his management had been so bad for so long.

## Lessons for risk management

The first and most important message is that good risk management depends on good clinical care. Risk assessment will never be an alternative to looking after the patient properly, and many of the failings in this case were in the basics of mental health care. Clunis's management was often careless in the literal sense of the word, i.e. without care. In much of his contact with hospitals there was no sense of the patient as a real human being, who needed looking after. Instead, professionals seemed to want to do the absolute minimum then be rid of him as soon as possible.

One standard for judging doctors and healthcare is the extent to which you would trust the service to look after one's mother, but in this case I had to shift the scale downward. If my dog did not get better follow-up care than this, I would find another vet.

**Table 3.1** Key facts about the mental health care of Christopher Clunis

1. His GP did not receive a single discharge summary or any communication from the mental health services involved in his care.

2. Although he had a caring and supportive family with whom he maintained contact throughout, services made no attempt to involve them in his care and they were never contacted when he was detained under the Mental Health Act 1983.

3. Services often referred to his drug use or the possibility of a drug-induced psychosis but there was never any evidence of drug use apart from his own assertions.

4. Much of what he said was unreliable, including claims to have been born in Sudan, married at the age of 2, and to have attended Eton, but services made little or no attempt to check the facts.

5. Clunis did well when he was on regular depot medication; he did badly when he was not.

6. He was discharged from hospital because of behavioural problems resulting from his mental illness and he was evicted from hostels for the same reason.

7. In the 4 years before the homicide he committed many violent offences but he was never convicted.

8. Clunis was not homeless when he first came into contact with services but became so because of his deteriorating mental state and a failure to help him.

9. The label of personality disorder was often applied to him but he had a normal personality before the onset of his schizophrenia.

10. Reports often failed to mention his growing history of violence and in some cases the omission was deliberate.

I make this point forcefully because it is important. Risk management begins not with checklists of risk factors and tables of statistics, but with a sense of caring about what happens to the patient when he walks out of the door of the clinic. Without that sense, the rest is a waste of time and energy. The whole point about risk is that it refers to the future rather than the here and now, so risk management is impossible if intervention considers only the present state.

The Clunis Inquiry agreed. There are positive comments among the list of criticisms and most are reserved for people who cared about the person they were looking after, while the most barbed criticism is directed at those professionals who could not wait to wash their hands of the case. Mistakes happen, and a lot can be forgiven if it arises in the context of trying to do one's best to help a patient. If, on the other hand, a service puts up the shutters after turning the patient away from the door, everyone involved had better be absolutely certain they got it right. Sympathy and excuses will be hard to find if it goes wrong.

A second major criticism was the failure to obtain background information. Historical risk factors for violence are no help if you have no history. It was not easy to get a history in this case, as the patient was often unco-operative and unreliable, but few professionals even tried. And there was no recognition of the deficiency. Few people expressed concern about the lack of background information. In some cases it is impossible to establish a history, but it is then necessary to acknowledge the deficiency and the consequent uncertainty. To act as if everything is known for certain is not only reckless but also arrogant.

Two aspects of the Clunis case illustrate this fault. Although they never set them out systematically, clinicians raised two diagnostic questions at several points. Was this presentation an episode of schizophrenia, or was it a drug-induced psychosis? And was this man's lack of co-operation a reflection of a personality disorder rather than mental illness? These questions arise frequently in mental health settings, and I deal with some of the general issues in Chapter 7. The main point in relation to Clunis was that there was never any serious attempt to address these questions. It may have been difficult to answer them but nobody even tried. There was occasional drug screening but clinicians did not mention the (negative) results. They were happy to go on speaking of a drug-induced psychosis even though there was never a positive drug screen or any direct evidence of drug use. Similarly, there was use of the term personality disorder without any attempt to get a proper history or to assess his personality.

Why do I find this so incredibly annoying? It is the abuse of medical power. Doctors get prestige and privileges from their scientific credentials. The scientific terms were used in the Clunis case to hide bad practice. Psychiatrists in the UK have to pass exams showing they understand statistics and can critically evaluate a scientific paper. Why bother, if their everyday practice amounts to spilling out pseudo-scientific terms with complete disregard for any supporting facts?

To make matters worse, one suspects the motivation was a desire to shift responsibility elsewhere. The unspoken coda to the diagnosis of personality disorder or drug-induced psychosis is '... so we do not have to look after him'.

## A digression: Clunis and capacity

It is impossible to resist the temptation to mention capacity at this point. In Chapter 1 I raised the hypothetical question of whether Clunis had capacity, and the implications of using a capacity test now become clear. The defence to some of the charges of bad practice would be that at the point of discharge Clunis had capacity, and he took the decision to leave and refuse further treatment. This may be workable in a service that was determined to provide optimum care to all patients against all obstacles, but it is disastrous if the service lacks the will or resources to provide more than the most rudimentary help. A capacity test in the Clunis case would have helped those staff whose main aim was a desire to wash their hands of all responsibility. For this reason alone, it is most unlikely that any politician who has read the Ritchie report will support the call for capacity-based mental health legislation. The fact that some psychiatrists have read it and still argue strongly for a capacity test just goes to show that professions have no shame when it comes to protecting their own interests.

## Short-term thinking

The Ritchie report identified the most serious failing as the absence of any long-term management plan to address Clunis's basic needs for care. Most service contacts were brief and often conveyed the impression that staff wanted to be rid of a problematic patient as quickly as possible. He was often discharged because he was violent on the ward, even though he was still psychotic. 'Risk management' here amounted to an attempt to get a high-risk patient out of the door as soon as possible.

When the Inquiry forced witnesses to address questions of risk, they were not impressed by the answers. One doctor said he had considered Clunis not to be a dangerous person because 'through all the threats of violence and waving knives there were just four abrasions to a hand recorded as actual injury'. By this time the patient had charged at police with a knife that it took three officers to remove from him; threatened to stab a fellow patient in the genital area; stabbed another patient when he was in bed at night with nursing staff intervening to prevent serious injury; and threatened to stab another patient in the eye. There had been numerous assaults not involving knives. The Inquiry concluded that the doctor's minimization of risk was 'misguided' and 'superficial' (ibid, p26).

It is credible that the poor risk assessment was due to lack of expertise but a more serious problem, and less easy to excuse, was a failure to disclose information about previous violence. Time and again reports omitted any mention of a history of violence, or even stated there was no such history. Again, this is all a world away from the theoretical limits of our ability to assess violence risk.

## Clunis in context

Although there were harsh comments about some of the staff involved, the main emphasis of the report was not on blame. It is impossible not to feel angry when one reads the Ritchie report and reflects on the unnecessary loss of one life, and the severe damage inflicted on several others. However, individual failings must be put in context, and much of the Ritchie report is about failings in service provision or organization. What made the case more depressing was a sense that this was simply how psychiatry was practiced, and that most psychiatrists would have behaved in the same way as the ones described. Resources were grossly inadequate, and a crucial recommendation was that London needed more secure psychiatric beds. It was also apparent that mental health services had been let down by the failure of the police to take action over Clunis's dangerous behaviour, and by the failure of the Crown Prosecution Service to press the case when he was in court.

I could dwell on these other failings, which deserve a book of their own. I choose not to dwell on them because this book is meant to assist people working in mental health. Most of them will not work in a perfect service, free of any resource constraints. Most of them will have to deal with a police force and prosecutors who have improved but are still too willing to leave mentally disordered offending to mental health services. In short, the world is neither perfect nor fair; working in it means living with its shortcomings.

Ethical practice in an imperfect world demands that services assess a patient's needs and decide on the best treatment, based on current knowledge. The next step is to implement the treatment plan as well as possible within resource constraints, and to document any restrictions and shortcomings. All too often, mental health services fail to follow this logic and mix up these decisions. The reasoning in the Clunis case sometimes appeared to progress as follows: I do not have enough beds; so I cannot say that the patient needs a bed; so I diagnose a condition that allows me not to recommend admission.

Such false logic is disastrous. It gives priority to the needs of the service over those of the patients, it conceals clinical need, and it makes it much more difficult to improve services because the shortcomings are never made explicit. It also puts clinicians in the firing line when things go wrong. The Clunis story could have been one of clinicians identifying need and arguing for more resources in a system stretched to breaking point. Instead it was a story of clinicians letting down their patient by denying his obvious needs, so taking the heat off the planners and politicians. Table 3.2 summarizes the correct and false logic involved, because this scenario is so common in mental health.

Note that the same logic applies in all branches of medicine but the false logic is easier to get away with in psychiatry because the problem or the need may be less obvious. If a man has a broken leg it is difficult to sustain the argument that it is only a bruise, whereas mental health services can often get away with the argument that schizophrenia is a drug-induced psychosis or malingering. The sad consequence is that mental health services often keep their own patients starved of resources. One of the commonest objections to better procedures for violence risk assessment is that services do not have the resources to support them. Clinicians in mental health seem to want to do the dirty work of politicians. Lack of resources may be the final verdict on any improvement in clinical care, but it should never be the first response.

**Table 3.2** Logic and false logic in clinical risk management

| Logic | False logic |
|---|---|
| 1. The patient needs intervention X | 1. Intervention X is not available |
| 2. Intervention X is not available | 2. There is no point recording the need for X |
| 3. Document the deficiency, give second best treatment | 3. Do something else |
| 4. Pressure on planners to meet the deficiency and consider buying X | 4. Planners never become aware of demand for X so service never improves |
| 5. Disaster arising from lack of X | 5. Disaster arising from lack of X |
| 6. Clinicians smell of roses. Planners have some explaining to do | 6. Planners smell of roses. Clinicians look incompetent |

The typical media story in physical medicine is very different. Clinicians discover newer, more effective treatments for cancer or heart disease; the health service goes pale and comes over all faint when it sees the cost; and there follows a debate with clinicians and patients on one side, demanding the best, and accountants and politicians on the other pointing out the fiscal realities. Mental health rarely gets to this stage because the clinicians start from the assumption they cannot afford to do things better. There is no better illustration of stigma in mental health and patients deserve more from those looking after them.

## The Falling Shadow

The basic facts of this story are soon told. A schizophrenic patient in an acute psychiatric unit stabbed and killed a female occupational therapist in 1993. The attack came without warning or interaction between perpetrator and victim. He was already detained as a civil patient under the Mental Health Act when he carried out the attack. The patient had unauthorized absences from the Unit, and it was during one of these absences that he bought the knife. He was not searched on his return to the hospital and the Inquiry was critical of lax procedures at the hospital, concluding that the homicide was not predictable but could probably have been prevented if policies had been followed correctly.

The story began 15 years earlier when the patient, then 21 years old, first became mentally ill while at college and developed an obsession with a fellow student after a brief relationship. Events came to a head when he stole a shotgun, held her hostage, and threatened to kill her. He was convicted of various offences and detained in Broadmoor high security hospital under a hospital order with restrictions, which were to be without limit of time. In other words, because of the gravity of the offence and the ongoing risk he posed to the public, the Home Secretary was to be given the final say on his transfer or discharge from hospital, and he could remain subject to indefinite, mandatory treatment and supervision after his conditional discharge back into the community.

The patient did well at Broadmoor because his illness responded readily to antipsychotic medication. Within 3 years he was transferred to a less secure hospital and a year after that he was home with his parents as a conditionally discharged patient. The main conditions on his discharge related to his continuing to receive psychiatric treatment. The doctors looking after him at Broadmoor were in no doubt that the improvement in his condition was due mainly to medication, so both his mental illness and the high risk of violence were likely to return if he stopped taking it.

In these circumstances, it may be difficult for outsiders to understand how the patient was able to stop all his medication within 3 years of returning to the community. Worse still, the psychiatrist supervising him recommended to a Mental Health Tribunal in 1986 that the patient should be discharged from the continuing restrictions on him, and the Tribunal followed that advice rather than the more cautious recommendations of the Home Office and the patient's social worker. From that point on, until the homicide, management was problematic, with psychotic relapses and poor compliance.

We are not dealing here with the theoretical limits of clinicians' ability to assess and manage risk, but with incompetence. There was a good risk-management plan in place when the patient left Broadmoor but the teams that looked after him in the community discarded it. How could this disaster (surely the correct term for such wilfully poor management, even without the homicide, which occurred 7 years later) happen?

The comforting explanation lies in blaming the individuals concerned, and some of them had little cause to complain when the Inquiry highlighted their mistakes. However, there are more general lessons to be learned.

First, psychiatrists have no faith in psychiatric treatment. They are so accustomed to giving patients medication that is flushed down the toilet, or produces only a partial response when it is taken, that they cannot recognize effective therapy when they see it. Time and time again, a patient with treated schizophrenia has his medication stopped because the doctor looking after him finds it easier to believe that that he never had schizophrenia in the first place, rather than accept that regular depot medication is keeping the disease under control. This patient did well on antipsychotic medication. The decision to stop it was about as sensible as stopping a diabetic's insulin because his condition is stable.

The second lesson is that psychiatrists are sometimes arrogant. The doctor who advised the Tribunal in this case had persuaded himself that the diagnosis was personality disorder rather than schizophrenia. He reached this conclusion without proper consideration of the alternative view and, in particular, without bothering to read the notes and reports relating to the patient's time at Broadmoor.

The Inquiry focused on later events and the extent to which the law allows early intervention to detain a patient under the civil provisions of the Mental Health Act. These are important questions but the civil parts of the Act were not designed to deal with long-term, continuing risks arising from a previous offence of serious violence. However carefully one fastened the stable door at a later date, the horse in this case had bolted long ago while the Tribunal was looking the other way.

### Comment

The reality of violence risk management in this case is a world away from theoretical worries about false positives and the statistical prediction of risk. Some clinicians are tempted to dismiss such cases as exceptions, but the sad truth is that Homicide Inquiries often feature misdiagnosis of schizophrenia as personality disorder, non-compliance with medication, and a failure to follow basic policies.

If the research on risk prediction told the whole story, we would expect to find in the Homicide Inquiries many accounts of mental health services pushing the outside of the envelope, struggling with the limits of their ability to predict or prevent violence. In this romantic vision the clinician is the radar operator squinting at a screen, trying to determine whether that vague blob is an enemy plane or a harmless flock of birds, but often let down by the inadequate technology of risk assessment.

Some Inquiry reports tell that story but most do not. It is more common to encounter failures to observe ordinary standards of clinical practice. A detained patient has unauthorized leave and is not searched on his return. Information is not passed on, to the extent that failures of communication have become a cliché of the Inquiries. Diagnoses and judgements are made on the basis of a single examination, with no consideration of previous assessments and records.

## The Jason Mitchell Inquiry

I use the name because it appears in the title of a book based on the Inquiry report (Blom-Cooper *et al.*, 1996). Readers interested in the full details of the case are referred to that book, or to a review (Maden, 1999). One of the main issues was again re-diagnosis as personality disorder of a man in whom the diagnosis of schizophrenia and associated risk of serious violence were well established. The misdiagnosis led to the omission of proper treatment. Apparent psychotic symptoms were explained away as the result of drug use, even though urine testing was never used to confirm that possibility.

### Comment

This Inquiry was a model of its kind and made the point that the homicides were not predictable and could not be understood in terms of any rational motivation. They were the product of highly abnormal thought processes resulting from a psychotic illness. On the one hand, there was some comfort to be derived from the fact that the outcome was not predictable, but on the other the inescapable message was that the killings would probably not have happened had the patient's mental illness been treated properly throughout its course rather than just in the early stages.

## Getting full value from the homicide Inquiries

It is only necessary to read a few Inquiries to detect the common themes running through them. Unfortunately, this information may not be readily available to clinicians. Two of the Inquiries above appeared as books, and book-length reports are common, even if they are not published as such. However penetrating the analysis, most clinicians are not going to read them because they have better things to do.

There have been attempts to review the Inquiries, with mixed success. The Zito Trust commissioned a compilation of the recommendations of the 54 Inquiries published between 1969 and 1996 (Sheppard, 1996). This publication, with the optimistic and well-intentioned title *Learning the Lessons*, amounted to a straight compilation of 750 or so bullet points. There was a lot of repetition of calls for better communication and better risk assessment, and the list was an odd mixture of the general and the specific.

Petch and Bradley (1997) reviewed *Learning the Lessons* and dealt with the problem of repetition by reducing the 750 points to a few themes. Prominent among them was the call for better training in risk assessment, but the authors do not take this recommendation any further. Most of the discussion in this paper is concerned with the overall impact of Inquiries on services. Most commentators in this area are more interested in the effects on staff than they are in the specific findings, which must be a great disappointment to outsiders. The paper ends on a defensive note, by claiming that it has not been established why psychiatric patients kill. Nevertheless '... many inquiries in their reports imply that there is something the psychiatric services can do to prevent this happening ... [but] ... This is far from certain ...'.

Some 10 years have passed since those words were written and they look even more defensive now. A small number of patients kill because they have schizophrenia, and an even smaller number of that group kill because their schizophrenia was not properly treated. Services can usually do something about this, and they will need to answer some tough questions if they cannot. Inquiries have made repeated calls for better assessment and management of violence risk, and the next three chapters look at ways in which services can improve their practice in this regard.

Chapter 7 returns to the Homicide Inquiries and consists mainly of an attempt to draw useful clinical lessons from a structured clinical analysis of some cases. It is an example of a different approach to a method that is becoming rather repetitive. However, the best example of a different approach to homicide Inquiries is the National Confidential Inquiry into Suicides and Homicides by patients with mental illness.

## A different approach to Homicide Inquiries

The UK National Confidential Inquiry into Suicide and Homicide by People with Mental Illness (NCISH) was established in 1996, in an attempt to overcome some of the problems associated with individual Inquiries. Its remit was to collect detailed clinical information on people who have had contact with specialist mental health services before committing suicide or homicide. It was modelled on other Confidential Inquiries, such as that into maternal deaths in childbirth, which are based on the assumption that confidentiality encourages clinicians to be open about mistakes that may have been made in the management of a case.

The combination of homicide and suicide reflects political and professional sensitivities and they are essentially separate Inquiries with different methodologies. Only the homicide Inquiry will be considered in detail here. Its aim was to collect detailed clinical information on those people convicted of a homicide who had any lifetime contact with mental health services, and to use that information to make recommendations for clinical practice and service provision.

The particular strength of the Confidential Inquiry is that is begins with a comprehensive sample of all homicides in the country, so the findings on mental disorder are placed in context. It represents a combination of good epidemiological research with the Inquiry method, so it has produced plenty of useful research in addition to the service recommendations.

## Methods used by the NCISH

The main database is a consecutive national series of patient homicides, where 'patient homicide' is defined as a homicide perpetrated by a person with life-time contact with mental health services. The definition is intentionally broad.

The three stages of data collection are as follows. First, details of all homicides are obtained from the Homicide Index maintained by the Home Office. Whenever possible the Inquiry obtains copies of psychiatric reports prepared for the trial as it is routine for there to be a report prepared in murder cases, even if there is no history of mental disorder.

The second stage is to send details of each case to mental health services in the offender's home area and adjacent areas, in order to identify those with a history of service contact. The trial reports provide an additional means of detecting mental health contacts. An offender becomes an Inquiry case whenever there has been such contact.

The third stage is to send a questionnaire to the consultant psychiatrist responsible for the patient's care, to obtain clinical and other information relating to the case. The questionnaire has both closed and open questions, so clinicians are invited to give their opinions on factors that may have contributed to the homicide, and factors that could have prevented it.

This method provides information about three groups of offenders: all homicide perpetrators; all those who had ever been in contact with mental health services; and those who had been in contact with services in the 12 months before the offence. For all perpetrators, the data collected include methods, victims and, for those with psychiatric reports, information on mental disorder and substance misuse at the time of the offence. For those with mental health contacts, the data include clinical history, details of care, events surrounding the killings, and opinions on prevention.

Although the methods of NCISH are scientific and the outputs include academic papers, the main output consists of reports designed to improve clinical practice. As an example of the approach, Table 3.3 lists the Inquiry's '12 Points to a Safer Service', some of which are concerned with the risk of self-harm.

As these points show, the Inquiry operates at a level of clinical detail that is not feasible in epidemiological studies. The cost is a loss of scientific precision, and the recommendations are a scientifically informed best guess rather than objective fact. In that respect they resemble most medical knowledge, even in the age of evidence-based practice, so we should not feel too embarrassed about an apparent lack of rigour. The recommendations go beyond the science into the area of clinical governance, reflecting the fact that the findings

**Table 3.3** Twelve points to a safer service (Appleby *et al.*, 2001)

| |
| --- |
| 1. Staff should receive training in the management of risk every 3 years |
| 2. All patients with severe mental illness and a history of self-harm or violence should receive the most intense level of care |
| 3. Individual care plans should specify action to be taken if the patient fails to attend or to comply with treatment |
| 4. There should be prompt access to services for patients in crisis and for their families |
| 5. Assertive outreach teams should be used to prevent loss of contact with vulnerable and high-risk patients |
| 6. Atypical antipsychotic medication should be available to all patients with severe mental illness who are non-compliant with 'typical' drugs because of side-effects |
| 7. There should be strategy for dual diagnosis patients covering training on the management of substance misuse, joint working with substance misuse services, and staff with specific responsibility to develop the local service |
| 8. In-patient wards should remove or cover all likely ligature points |
| 9. There should be follow-up within 7 days of discharge from hospital for everyone with severe mental illness or a history of self-harm in the previous 3 months |
| 10. Patients with a history of self-harm in the last 3 months should receive supplies of medication covering no more than 2 weeks |
| 11. There should be local arrangements for sharing information with criminal justice agencies |
| 12. There should be a policy of post-incident multidisciplinary case review and the information should be given to families of involved patients |

are concerned not with cold, clinical observations but with matters of life and death. Yet again, we are reminded of the values bearing on these topics, and the way they shape research and practice.

The key findings on homicides are summarized in Table 3.4, which combines data from Appleby *et al.* (1999, 2001) and Shaw *et al.* (2004, 2006).

## We have a problem … the NCISH findings

The findings are broadly consistent with other sources and confirm that mental illness is involved in a small but significant proportion of homicides in England and Wales. Mentally ill perpetrators are less likely to be involved in stranger homicides, in which the typical perpetrator is a young man who has been drinking or using drugs (Shaw *et al.*, 2004).

The message to the public is reassuring in terms of the relative risk of homicide represented by mental illness, but the figures pose more difficult questions for those involved in mental health. The headline figure is surely the 5% prevalence of schizophrenia among perpetrators of homicide, compared with

**Table 3.4** Key findings on homicide in England and Wales from the National Confidential Inquiry into Suicide and Homicide (NCISH)

---

◆ 10% of perpetrators receive a verdict of manslaughter on the grounds of diminished responsibility or infanticide

◆ Over half the men but only one-fifth of women are convicted of murder

◆ The prevalence of schizophrenia in homicide perpetrators is 5%

◆ At final service contact, immediate and long-term risk of violence were estimated to be low in over 75% of cases

◆ Mental health teams considered that 17% of relevant homicides were preventable

◆ 59% of respondents were able to identify factors that would have reduced risk, particularly better compliance, closer supervision and better contact with the patient's family

◆ Of patients in recent contact with services, over one-fifth were non-compliant with drug treatment in the month before the offence

---

its 1% prevalence in the general population. These population figures are consistent with Taylor and Gunn's (1984) findings in remanded prisoners, and there is no reason to doubt the validity of the association.

It would be wrong to jump to conclusions and there may be several causes for this association. For example, social and personal factors predisposing to violence may be associated with schizophrenia, so the causal link is indirect. Even when the violence was a consequence of the mental illness, it may have been impossible to prevent because the illness presented with violence, or because the killing happened despite optimum treatment. But these explanations should not obscure the likelihood that better management of the mental illness would have prevented some of these deaths—not all of them, but more than enough to make the exercise of better risk management worthwhile.

The other findings of NCISH support this possibility, suggesting that risk assessment was often inaccurate, and that the homicide could usually have been prevented (see also Chapter 7). The inescapable conclusion is that inadequate violence risk management is contributing to the over-representation of patients with schizophrenia among perpetrators of homicide.

A brave and ambitious service would set itself the target of reducing that 5% figure over the next 5–10 years, through better risk management.

## Homicide Inquiries in the future

There will continue to be a role for independent Inquiries, when the circumstances of a particular case are such as to indicate a special public interest. In general, such Inquiries are unlikely to lead to further service improvements.

The future lies with the more systematic combination of rigorous research methodology applied to relevant clinical questions, as in the NCISH.

While further knowledge will emerge from NCISH and similar approaches to the problem, the major issue for services is not new knowledge but the implementation of what we already know. The case for wider use of structured clinical assessment of violence risk is overwhelming.

Chapter 4

# Clinical assessment of violence risk

## Introduction

The three options for assessing violence risk are:

1. unstructured clinical assessment
2. standardized or actuarial assessment
3. structured clinical assessment.

These models are sometimes referred to as first, second, or third generation, but there is no advantage to these terms. The headings above are descriptive and short enough for routine use. Also, the notion of first, second, and third generations implies progression or evolution, whereas all three may be in use at the same time. In fact, the same clinician may make use of all these methods for different purposes.

The present chapter deals with unstructured clinical assessment. Chapter 5 covers standardized and actuarial methods, while Chapter 6 sets out the structured clinical approach. Inevitably the emphasis is on the differences but they also have a lot in common. While structured clinical assessment has advantages as an overall approach and is 'the best' if one has to choose, the others have their place and value.

## Risk and history

The best predictor of violence is previous violence

*The Second Law of Forensic Psychiatry*

The irritating thing about the statement above is that, like many aphorisms, it has a core of inescapable truth but does not tell the whole story. Monahan (1981) expressed similar sentiments in a more general statement: '... if there is one finding that overshadows all others in the area of prediction, it is that the probability of future crime increases with each prior criminal act'. Yet life is more complicated and we know that offending tends to decrease with age from about 25 years on, so the probability of crime is not always rising as the individual offends.

The message for clinicians is that any attempt to assess violence risk must include reference to previous violence but the method cannot rely exclusively on what has gone before. This is actually good news. It would be dispiriting to think we can hope to manage violence risk only after violence has already happened. Risk management may be more difficult when there is no history of violence, but it is certainly possible. Conversely, even when there is an extensive history of violence, future violence is not inevitable.

The core of real truth in the aphorism is that risk management requires a full description and understanding of any previous violence. This chapter and the next two deal with the assessment of violence risk. The methods differ in the degree of structure, but they are all based in part on a description of the past. That description includes factors that are generally associated with increased violence risk, such as psychopathy and mental illness. It may also include factors linked to actual or threatened violence in the specific patient, and these may be general (mental illness and relapse) or idiosyncratic (he argues with his father, or he does not like Mondays). The aim is to understand how violence came about, and so to predict conditions that will make violence more or less likely in the future.

The flaw in this reasoning is that there is a first time for everything. People may be more or less creatures of habit, but all have moments of innovation or inspiration. The essence of the notion of a criminal career is that it involves change, development and, in some cases, escalation. This is not an argument for abandoning all attempts to assess risk, but we need to be aware of our limitations. We can make statements about whether people are more or less likely to be violent, and under what circumstances, but there will always be room for surprises. In fact, the notion of surprise is crucial in evaluating actuarial methods, and it will be discussed further in Chapter 5.

## Unstructured clinical assessment of violence risk: anarchists and gurus

In its purest form the clinical method is the anarchist's version of risk assessment because it has no rules. The clinician is free to collect any information, to combine and process it in any way, and to state the conclusions in any form. The credibility of the assessment derives not from any scientific method or scheme, but from the credentials and reputation of the expert concerned. So this method is favoured by men in three-piece suits and half-moon glasses; unlikely gurus, perhaps, but they have the same reliance on charismatic

**Table 4.1** Disadvantages of unstructured clinical assessment of risk

| |
| --- |
| No evidence base |
| Reliance on charismatic authority |
| Difficult to challenge—or defend |
| Low reliability |
| Low validity |
| Susceptible to counter-transference |
| Susceptible to bias and prejudice |

authority. They are right because of who they are, and the classic response to challenge is: 'And who are you?' The disadvantages of this method are obvious but for completeness they are listed in Table 4.1.

The main argument in favour of this method is that experienced clinicians may be good at it, but that advantage is outweighed by the lack of transparency. Even if the risk assessment is accurate it is impossible to know how the decision was reached, so it is difficult to question it. Lack of transparency leaves the method wide open to allegations of discrimination on ethnic or other grounds. With a patient's liberty at stake this is no way to proceed in a civilized and democratic society, so most clinical assessments incorporate a degree of structure.

In its most basic form, the structure derives from the training of the professionals involved. Doctors tend to collect similar data and to present it in the conventional form of family history, followed by personal history, leading on to mental state examination, and ending with conclusions. There are still no rules about how the conclusion is derived from the material that has gone before, but the basic structure makes it easier for other professionals to check the data and to gain some understanding of how the conclusions were reached.

Most professionals are taught to express their opinions in terms of risk rather than dangerousness, so here too structure is creeping in to clinical assessments. In fact, it is probably fair to say that true, unstructured assessment of violence risk is no longer an acceptable method, so we are really dealing with degrees of structure.

A good example of this approach is Gunn's (1993) framework for clinical risk assessment. Gunn is not an enthusiast for structured or standardized assessment but presents a framework to guide clinical practice, which can be adapted to a range of situations. The main headings are presented in Table 4.2.

The immediate response may be that this is simply a description of the steps necessary for a full clinical assessment. And so it is, but there is nothing wrong in that. We need to demystify the process of risk assessment and management,

**Table 4.2** A framework for clinical risk assessment (from Gunn, 1993)

| |
| --- |
| Detailed life history |
| Substance abuse |
| Psychosexual assessment |
| Description of previous offending/antisocial behaviour |
| Psychological assessments |
| Mental state assessments |
| Attitude to treatment/insight |

and to recognize that much of the time it is good clinical practice given a new spin. To illustrate the nature of that spin, it is helpful to expand on some of the headings and to show how they relate to violence risk.

1. *Detailed life history*. This should begin with a family history, including mental disorder, substance misuse and criminality in other family members. Mental disorder includes personality disorder and, while it is difficult to ask directly about it, descriptions of parental behaviour provide plenty of clues. We tend to forget that heredity accounts for between about one quarter and two thirds of the determination of personality, so a family history provides a strong pointer to the diagnosis. A fuller assessment will use other informants or records, including medical or social services reports dealing with the parents.

   The developmental history should include experience of neglect, abuse, or disruption in childhood, as well as educational attainment and disciplinary problems at school or at home. A history of conduct disorder or delinquency is important; about half of all conduct-disordered children grow up to have a personality disorder in adulthood. One of the most useful distinctions is between adolescence-limited or life-course-persistent delinquency (Moffitt, 1993), the latter being highly predictive of personality disorder.

   The adult history should include occupational, social, and leisure activities. A full account includes the time spent in different jobs, reasons for changing jobs, and details of any periods of unemployment.

2. *Substance abuse history*. A description of drug and alcohol misuse should include age of onset, course, symptoms of dependency, funding of habit, experience of treatment, current state, associated offending and social or behavioural problems.

3. *Psychosexual assessment*. The extent of this assessment will depend on the particular case. It is wrong to expect intimate details at a first interview

and a full exploration of this topic may have to wait. In some sexual offenders, the obtaining of a full psychosexual history is so difficult that it could be set as a treatment goal.

A full history includes development of sexual awareness, experience of puberty, any history of sexual abuse as a child or an adult, and exploration of any aberrant sexual interests and fantasies, including the presence of misogyny.

Although a detailed psychosexual assessment may emerge only late in assessment or treatment, a basic relationship history is an essential part of any violence risk assessment. The basic history of relationships should include duration, reasons for ending, occurrence of violence, and contact with any children.

4. *Description of previous offending or antisocial behaviour.* This description should begin with childhood problems and include all antisocial behaviour, whether or not it led to prosecution. In offenders one should note dates of convictions, the patient's own account of the offences (to be compared with other records when possible), the sentences imposed, the patient's attitude towards the offence, and his attitude towards any victims.

In patients with long histories of offending it is important to consider the balance between time spent in and out of custody, which may identify individuals who are unable to survive in the outside world for more than a short period. They represent a high risk of future offending, although not necessarily future violence. Behaviour within custody is also important and can shed light on peer relationships and attitudes to authority.

5. *Psychological assessments.* They may include IQ or personality measures as appropriate. Low intelligence has a weak but significant association with offending and it will also influence the type of intervention that may be appropriate.

Standardized measures of personality may be useful but most rely on self-report, so they are not to be relied upon in precisely those individuals who cause most concern. In such cases the criminal record may be a better guide to personality than information obtained from self-report or interview.

Exceptions to this rule include the Personality Assessment Schedule (Tyrer 2000) and the Psychopathy Checklist—Revised (PCL-R, Hare, 1991). The first makes use of informants and the second requires the use of records, including criminal records. The latter has been extensively validated in both prison and forensic psychiatric populations and should be completed in all suspected high-risk offenders.

Standardized or actuarial risk assessment instruments may be relevant in forensic populations (see Chapter 5).

6. *Assessments of mental state.* The emphasis is on serial assessments of mental state over time, with recognition that a single assessment may be misleading. One should also include assessments of mental state at other times, particularly during previous offending, based on the accounts of patient, relatives/informants, and police or court records as appropriate. Witness statements, including those of victims when available, are essential if there has been serious violent offending. Such statements may shed valuable light on the offender's mental state at the time of the offence.

7. *Attitude to treatment and insight.* Does the patient see himself as suffering from any form of mental disorder, and in need of any sort of help? Does he see previous treatment as having been helpful? Did he cooperate with it? Does he express remorse for previous antisocial behaviour, and does he make a connection between that behaviour and mental disorder?

## Collecting information

This framework is adaptable to all situations, and it must be adapted. A detailed exploration of sexuality will not be welcomed by the middle-aged clergyman with a spot of depression, whereas it is essential in the assessment of a young man alleged to have harassed women. In either case, an initial interview is not the best situation in which to get the information.

One should assume that the interview with the patient provides an assessment of the mental state, whereas the history comes from independent sources. This is too cynical a view for ordinary psychiatric practice, and one rarely has the luxury of sufficient independent information to establish a full history. Still, one should always be aware of the assumptions involved in taking a patient's account at face value. That account may be true in most cases, but you have no right to be surprised if it turns out to be false. It is, of course, in the nature of things that deceit is most likely on those occasions when it matters most. The motivation to conceal is strongest in those who have something to hide, and the ability to deceive is most highly developed in some psychopaths. It is also important to detect deceit because it has implications for future treatment, supervision, and monitoring.

## Recording and communication of information

At the risk of making a mantra out of a cliché, there is no getting around the fact that risk management is impossible without good records. If in doubt, write it down. There are few certainties in psychiatry, so most decisions can be defended if there is a record of having considered alternatives, setting out the reasons for adopting one course of action rather than another.

The sharing of information with others requires good records but written communication is no substitute for face to face meetings. It is easy to see such meetings as necessary compliance with Government guidelines, while forgetting the reasons for their importance.

Good communication requires support structures, the most important being a clinical information system. It is an indictment of the NHS that such systems are a rarity in psychiatric practice; and it is an indictment of the English independent Homicide Inquiries that they rarely mention this problem, despite an obsession with individual failures of communication.

## Making sense of the data

It is easy but wrong to reduce risk assessment to a process of collecting information. There will always remain the question of what to do with that information. The process is based on three assumptions:

1. *There is consistency in the behaviour of an individual over time.* This assumption is necessary as, without some consistency, any prediction becomes impossible. It is the basis of the maxim 'the best predictor of violence is previous violence'. By defining the circumstances in which violence has occurred in the past, including its motivations and relationship to mental disorder, we hope to identify future risks.

2. *Some characteristics, other than previous violence, increase the probability of future violence.* These characteristics include substance misuse and certain personality disorders. They are important as they allow the assessment of risk in people who have not yet been violent.

3. *Detailed knowledge of a person increases the chances of predicting behaviour.* The best evidence for this assertion is that we are not continually surprised by the behaviour of our friends. In general, they react to life in a way that is broadly consistent with our image of them.

These assumptions allow the organization of the data we have collected about an individual, in order to formulate a risk assessment and management plan. It should specify:

1. the nature of the risk, i.e. of what and to whom?

2. the extent of the risk

3. warning signs

4. factors likely to increase the risk

5. factors likely to decrease the risk

6. contingency plans.

Note that this structure is similar to that used in describing the feared scenarios of violence in the HCR20 (Historical Clinical Risk-20; Chapter 6). It is reassuring that, despite all the arguments over precisely how to measure violence risk, there is a common thread running through much of the work in this area.

Management decisions will be taken on the basis of the formulation above. Even with the formulation, there is still a massive gap between the information collected and the decision. The risk assessment does not tell us what to do, and we need clinical judgement to cross the gap between information and decision.

## Clinical judgement, team working, and second opinions

Clinical judgement has been much maligned because doctors have sometimes used it to discourage any scrutiny of their actions. It can be a screen behind which clinicians hide, and when used in that way it deserves all the bad press. At worst it is another way of saying that doctor knows best.

On the other hand, so long as there are uncertainties within medicine, we cannot live without clinical judgements. We need to rehabilitate this concept, in its proper place, if medicine is to survive and prosper as a scientifically respectable occupation. Clinical judgement is one of the (many) things that distinguish medicine from chemistry or physics, and it is misleading to pretend there can ever be complete certainty or accuracy. The field of mental heath involves more than the average amount of clinical judgement, because there are fewer certainties. The surgeon can confirm that a bone is broken when he sees it on an X-ray, but the psychiatrist will rarely have such luxury. Risk assessment in mental health is all about making better-informed clinical judgements.

This theme is developed in the next chapter, which considers actuarial risk assessment as a doomed attempt to do away with clinical judgement. Assuming for now that we have to use clinical judgement, we can consider the safeguards that should surround it, and the most important of these is consultation with others. The point is that there is no right answer, so sensible decisions are more likely if they are based on a wide range of knowledge and opinion.

Those consulted may include the patient, relatives, carers or other interested parties. In cases where the risk is high, clinicians may refer decisions to courts, tribunals or the Home Office/Justice Department. In these high-risk cases, referral to another authority may improve decision-making but it is also right in principle: we are not dealing with purely medical decisions, and clinicians should not take upon themselves either the full authority or the full responsibility. This principle is discussed below, when considering a model for risk management.

Consultation with colleagues warrants special consideration. I have already said that most psychiatric decisions can be defended if there is a written record of having considered various alternatives. I will now go a stage further and argue that all decisions can be defended if other clinicians have endorsed them. Multidisciplinary team working is an example of this process, and the clichés are all true: a trouble shared is a trouble halved, and two heads are better than one, etc. When making complex decisions, teams do a better job than individuals acting alone.

The underlying assumption is that the multidisciplinary team is working effectively. All members of the team must feel able to voice their opinions, debate the issue freely, then arrive at a collective decision they can support. There is no point in having a team if you do not listen to what they say, or if you ignore it all the time.

In contentious cases it is helpful to go outside the team to seek a second opinion. In matters of clinical judgement the final arbiter is the opinion of one's peers so you may as well ask them for their views before taking the decision, rather than having them give opinions to an Inquiry later. At best the second opinion will offer new insights and a better strategy for managing the case, and at worst it provides an endorsement for the existing management plan.

## Clinical judgement, science, and the future

Clinical judgement is indispensable to risk management in mental health. It may occupy that position for want of a better alternative, but it should always be informed by science. Most recent developments are in numerical and standardized measures, which are considered in the following chapter. Before moving on, it is important to acknowledge some general principles relating to medical expertise and authority. Medicine derives its credibility from science, which is a stronger base than many other fields of knowledge can claim, but it has limits.

Failure to recognize the limits of science leads to misuses of medical power, in which doctors give opinions on matters in which they have no expertise. This is never good. First, the public is increasingly intolerant of the arbitrary exercise of professional power. Second, power and responsibility tend to go together. Those who pontificate on matters beyond their expertise cannot complain when they are held responsible for matters over which they have no control. As scrutiny and criticism of practice increases, mental health workers need to have a clear idea of the questions they can and cannot be expected to address. It is easier to understand this problem if risk management is broken down into its three component parts.

## A three-stage model of risk management

The process of assessing and managing the risk of violence has the following components:

1. What is the nature and extent of the risk?
2. To what extent can the risk be reduced by treatment?
3. Is the residual risk acceptable?

These three stages are implicit in mental health work, even though we are not used to breaking down the risk assessment process into these separate tasks. So why bother to separate them now? The answer emerges when we consider each process in turn.

### What is the nature and extent of the risk?

Once we accept that violence is a complication in some cases of mental disorder, this is an appropriate question for the psychiatrist or other expert. Courts, Tribunals, and other bodies are entitled to expect that mental health workers will have specialist knowledge of the relationship between violence and mental disorder. While the level of skill varies between individual practitioners, there are accepted techniques of risk assessment.

Note that this argument is not about the level of accuracy, where there is plenty of room for debate and improvement. Nor am I suggesting that expert evidence should be accepted uncritically. There will always be room for differences of opinion and for debate but such disputes should not obscure the principle, that this is the legitimate domain of the mental health practitioner.

### To what extent can the risk be reduced by treatment?

Again, while the expert may be unable to answer this question accurately, it is reasonable to ask. Who else should answer such a question, if not someone who earns a living by treating mental disorder? There may be formidable technical and practical problems, but the enterprise is a legitimate one.

### Is the residual risk acceptable?

The third question differs from the others in that it is not the business of an expert. Why should a doctor decide on the level of risk that is acceptable to an individual, or to a group? Medical training does not enable one to answer a question of this type, and it could never do so, because it is not that sort of question. People are capable of deciding for themselves on the level of risk they are prepared to accept. They are (rightly) suspicious of any professional group that attempts to take over that function, even though they may ask experts for advice on the extent of the risk.

Smoking is a good example. We want advice from doctors on the nature and extent of the risks involved, and we may want to know how we can reduce those risks, but we want to decide for ourselves whether or not to light up.

This is a difficult area for medicine, which tends always towards paternalism. It is understandable that watching people die of cancer should result in a desire to prohibit the use of tobacco, and that awareness of the brain's fragility leads to calls for a ban on boxing. The public expect doctors to preach and to campaign on such issues, but they have no sympathy for professionals who impose their will on others. People like to take their own decisions about risk.

## Optimism and realism: the philosophy of violence risk management

The clinical approach to violence risk management consists of the methods of ordinary clinical practice put to a different use, or given a different emphasis. Good risk assessment differs from good clinical practice because of the context, or the background assumptions. Risk assessment depends on an awareness that things can, and do, go wrong.

One of the problems here is that, as noted in previous chapters, the risk of serious violence in psychiatry is not generally very high. A clinician can go through a whole career with fingers crossed and head in the sand, yet never run into problems as a result of a serious assault by a patient. But even if the odds are not too bad, this is still reckless gambling. The essence of risk management is to discard the assumption that nothing can go wrong, and to foresee the possibility that luck alone may not be enough to guard against disaster.

A philosophical shift of this type can be difficult for clinicians because medical training tends to emphasize a positive message in the face of adversity. We know that most diseases are incurable and we know that everybody dies, but medical services emphasize hope and motivation. This is a good and inevitable thing. Cheery optimism and happy endings will always be more popular choices in the hospital library than Thomas Hardy or Samuel Beckett. However, clinicians should be careful not to believe their own propaganda. Things can and do go wrong, and we do patients a disservice if we fail to recognize the possibility of disaster.

By contrast with the habitual optimism of medical practice, the life insurance industry survives and thrives only by reminding us of our mortality, and by making hard-headed and accurate estimates of its limits. The next chapter considers standardized or actuarial methods of risk assessment, which have attempted to apply the methods of life insurance to the more complicated area of violence risk assessment.

## Summary: unstructured clinical assessment of violence risk

The heyday of unstructured risk assessment was a time when experts derived authority from who they were, rather than from what they did. That era passed with the advent of closer scrutiny and better governance, and few mourned its demise. Professionals are subject to better regulation and closer scrutiny, so even unstructured risk assessments involve a minor degree of structure. The best include all the information that is incorporated in more formal schemes.

Whatever the precise method used, it is necessary to recognize the limits to medical expertise, so as to avoid being held responsible for things over which one has no control.

One of the key principles of risk management is a willingness to accept that things can and do go wrong, which is the first step in contingency planning.

# Chapter 5

# Standardized or actuarial risk assessment

In this life we want nothing but Facts, sir; nothing
but facts.

> Thomas Gradgrind, *Hard Times* by Charles Dickens

Just the facts, Ma'am. Just the facts.

> Sgt Joe Friday, *Dragnet*

The previous chapter showed that unstructured clinical judgement has many limitations as a way of estimating violence risk. Most people agree that clinical risk assessment is improved by systematic data collection and recording, and there is probably a general consensus as to the type of information that should be collected. Everybody agrees on the importance of knowing about previous violence; substance misuse, non-compliance, lack of insight, and personality disorder. Given such agreement, the obvious next step is to consider whether such factors can be included in a systematic assessment that offers a superior alternative to clinical judgement.

This is a tempting, even seductive prospect. Unlike the old concept of dangerousness, risk lends itself to a systematic, statistical approach. We can describe and measure specific risks, the most common being violent and sexual offending. Once we attach a probability to these risks, we open up all sorts of possibilities for statistical manipulation. The most important of these possibilities is standardization, allowing us to compare a patient with a population and conjuring up visions of benchmarks, yardsticks, and all those other trappings of physics from which psychological scientists seek to borrow credibility and respectability.

This chapter describes the origins and techniques of standardized risk assessment. It explains both the power of standardized techniques and the limitations—which are considerable.

Two analogies are particularly useful in understanding standardized risk assessment. The first is with the life insurance industry, which relies for its success on accurate, if limited, predictions about the future. The second analogy is with IQ testing, probably the most well developed example of a standardized psychological test. These comparisons illustrate both the strengths and the limitations of standardized risk assessment.

It is easier to understand the problems in this area by referring to specific examples, and I make particular use of the Violence Risk Appraisal Guide (VRAG; Harris *et al.*, 1993) for this purpose. I use it as an example because it is widely used and easy to understand. It is one of the best actuarial measures, and the problems it reveals are mostly limitations of the general approach rather than defects of this particular scale.

One of the most important messages of this chapter is that the actuarial approach has fundamental and unavoidable limitations, which are unrelated to the particular items used in a scale. It follows logically that these problems cannot be overcome by creating a newer and better actuarial scale because they are intrinsic to this way of looking at the world.

## Actuarial risk assessment: insurance salesmen and boffins

> *Actuary:* a person who compiles and analyses statistics in order to calculate insurance risks and premiums. (Derived from the Latin: *actus*, event or thing done, and *actuarius*, bookkeeper).

The derivation of the word helps in understanding the process. The basic technique is a careful recording of events and actions. It is history. The actuary describes what happened in the past then predicts the future on the assumption that it will be a replay of what has gone before. There is no underlying theory or explanation. The actuarial method claims to tell it like it is—or like it was, at any rate. There is no interest in the how or why, but only in the facts.

This approach has a down-home, no nonsense appeal. Why worry about complicated theories of offending behaviour when you can go for the plain facts? If history tells us that economic deprivation was associated with offending, we should base our future plans on the assumption that deprived areas will have higher than average rates of offending, with no need to worry about the reasons for that association. History also tells us that psychopathy and childhood conduct disorder are associated with violent offending, so we can safely predict an increased risk when those features are present.

Insurance companies depend for their survival on reliable information of this kind. They apply data to groups, in order to determine insurance premiums. Smokers pay more for their life insurance because they are more likely to die.

People living in inner cities pay more for their household insurance because they suffer high crime rates. These facts do not mean that any individual living in a town will be a victim of burglary or that all rural dwellers will be safe. They do not mean that all non-smokers live longer. But so long as the differences between groups are maintained in the long run, insurance companies can make a profit. Insurance companies rely on group projections, but they are not in the business of individual prediction—unlike mental health workers, who do care what happens to individual patients. It is here that the limitations of the actuarial method become apparent.

Take the example of ethnic origin and imprisonment. In England and Wales, there are about 46 million people over the age of 10 years, of whom 1.38 million (3%) are classified as of black ethnic origin. When the prison population of England and Wales was about 60 000, it included 7200 people (12%) classified as black. The odds ratio for black ethnic origin and imprisonment is therefore 4.41, with a 95% confidence interval of 4.3–4.52. In lay terms, black people are about four times more likely to find themselves in prison, compared with people of other ethnic groups.

This statistical association is stronger than that between smoking and lung cancer, so the actuary cannot afford to ignore it. The arguments about causation are irrelevant. If the company offered insurance against imprisonment, black people would be paying more. Most people with even a trace of liberal or humanist sensibility will find this approach deeply troubling. It is a classic example of stereotyping or prejudice, in which people are treated not as individuals but as members of a class.

And it gets worse. The next step is to assume that the probabilities apply to the individual sitting in front of you. If we conclude that he is more likely to be a criminal because of the colour of his skin, the errors in reasoning become overt racism. We reject such an approach out of hand. Yet actuarial measures, applied to individual patients, rely on precisely the same reasoning. The actuarial method describes the behaviour of a group or class to which our patient belongs, whether that group is psychopaths, schizophrenics, or drug addicts, then assumes the patient will behave in the same way. It is not surprising that some US courts have rejected actuarial risk assessment on the grounds that it is not a clinical assessment. In fact, it is not truly an individual assessment at all.

Clinicians can be forgiven at this point for wanting to ditch the standardized or actuarial approach. They should not be so impulsive. There is a perfectly good baby drowning in that dirty bathwater. Actuarial tools have value in providing a context for individual, clinical assessment, so long as they are not used to replace it. Other branches of medicine do not embark on clinical assessment without bearing in mind the background risks, and mental health should be no different.

Also, for all the claims of relying only on the observed facts, many actuarial instruments turn out to be grounded in well-established research findings. Most of the items that make up the VRAG might have been chosen from a reading of the literature, even though the scale was not constructed in that way. As a result, actuarial measures provide a useful summary of background risk factors. I return to this point below when discussing psychopathy, which underpins many standardized risk assessments, but first it is necessary to consider actuarial measures of violence risk in more detail. How do they compare with other standardized psychological tests?

## IQ tests and standardization: the instant expert

The thread running through this chapter is the tension between the individual and the group. We can describe how groups of people have behaved in the past, but it is not a straightforward matter to apply this knowledge to the individual.

The tension between group facts and individuals is not unique to risk assessment, or to standardized scales. It runs through the whole of clinical practice. The value of experience is that the experienced clinician has seen many different patients so has a feel for where the new patient sits in relation to them. The expert assessment of an individual case has something in common with actuarial assessment, in that it depends on the expert's knowledge of a large group of patients. The difference is that the expert assessment leaves room for discretion in which background facts to use, and how to evaluate them. One of the problems is that it takes time to acquire experience, and everyone wants to be the patient of the experienced clinician rather than the doctor who is still racking up the clinical mileage.

Standardization offers a way out of this dilemma by providing instant access to more experience than can be obtained in a lifetime of clinical practice. Once a test or measure is standardized, a person's score can be compared with that of a population and we can see precisely where that patient fits on the spectrum or bell-shaped curve. There is no need for the person carrying out the assessment to have had vast clinical experience, because the background knowledge has been incorporated into the test.

The best example within psychology is IQ (Intelligence Quotient) as a measure of intelligence. An experienced teacher can assess a pupil's academic potential in a reasonably short time, but an intelligence test is quicker. The test is designed so the average score in the population is 100, and learning difficulties are defined as beginning below 70. The IQ score of an individual places him in relation to these standards. If the score is 60 he may need help from services for those with learning difficulties. If the score is 120 he will probably do well in school and may go to university.

The use of IQ as an alternative to professional expertise illustrates the appeal of the standardized approach to managers, planners, and accountants. Why deal with experienced professionals, with all the associated costs and personal quirks, when a technician can use a test to do the same job?

## From IQ to violence risk: the limits of testing

Standardized or actuarial assessments such as the VRAG extend this approach to the measurement of violence risk. Instead of academic achievement they are concerned with violent or sexual offending, but the statistical principles are similar. We know how scores or features are distributed in the population, and we locate the individual in relation to that population.

There is an apparent difference between IQ and violence risk in that IQ tests measure performance in the here and now, whereas risk assessment is concerned with offending in the future. In reality, both have elements of prediction. The WAIS (Wechsler Adult Intelligence Scale) and other IQ tests are valuable not because we need to know how well a person does on that test, but because we expect the WAIS score to predict future performance. Also, the predicted performance can be generalized. IQ tests would be of limited use if they predicted only performance on IQ tests, and they have become accepted because they predict broader academic performance.

Intelligence testing has stood the test of time because it is a reasonably accurate predictor of individual performance in a particular area, but it is not perfect. Some of these imperfections apply to risk assessment or any other standardized test so it is worth looking at them in more detail.

1. **Testing problems.** The individual may have an off-day when tested, in which case future performance will be better than the result predicts. In risk assessment errors of this type are most likely to occur because of incomplete or inaccurate recording of historical information. There may be a lack of reliable information about disturbed behaviour in childhood, or offending behaviour may have gone undetected or escaped prosecution. Conversely, violence related to circumstantial factors may elevate an actuarial score where it will appear to reflect characteristics of the individual.

2. **Failure to generalize.** If future tasks have little in common with the IQ test, the score will be a less accurate predictor of performance. For example, some people with a high IQ perform poorly on tasks requiring good empathy and social skills. Actuarial measures of risk may fail to pick up

specific risk factors for violence, related to circumstances such as a tempestuous relationship.

3. **Change over time**. IQ is fairly stable but it does change, and it may change dramatically if cognitive function declines as a result of disease, drugs, or trauma. This may seem a trivial point in relation to IQ but it is a massive problem with actuarial risk assessment. A high-risk patient may become much less of a risk as he grows older or his mental illness is treated, and he may suddenly become less of a risk if incapacitated by physical illness. There are a host of less obvious changes in risk that relate to dynamic risk factors such as stress or substance misuse.

4. **Uneven performance**. IQ is a measure of general intelligence but cognitive function can be patchy. The autistic individual with general learning difficulties but islands of exceptional performance has become a cliché. Many people have specific talents that are not reflected in an IQ score, so they do better in life than testing would predict. Others have specific weaknesses that mean task performance does not live up to the expectations created by the IQ test. Within a large population none of this matters much, because it all evens out and IQ remains a good overall predictor. At the level of the individual these variations are crucial, and it would be unwise to choose anyone for a job on the basis of intelligence alone. The problem is even worse in risk assessment, and it is common for there to be individual, idiosyncratic factors that render any general risk assessment null and void. A monosymptomatic delusion, or morbid jealousy, may indicate a high risk of violence even when all other indicators are favourable, and this fact alone should steer us away from relying solely on any actuarial assessment of violence risk.

Risk assessment is less well-established than IQ testing and it does not have the same precision or stability, but both measures grapple with the same underlying issue of using past performance to predict future behaviour in different but related situations. There is room for error in IQ testing because of the gap between past and future, and the potential for error is greater in violence risk management because more variables have a bearing on the outcome.

Actuarial risk assessment has one advantage over IQ testing, in that it is mainly reliant on what the patient has done in the past, rather than what he says at interview or how he performs on a pencil and paper test. Assuming one can get the history correct, data on previous offending and violence are as hard as data get in the notoriously soft world of psychological testing, which is so often reliant on self-report.

At this point it is necessary to look critically at the possibility of ever predicting the future. It is here that the insurance industry has most to teach clinicians, but the most important lesson is about the limitations of the method. There is no such thing as a crystal ball, and the type of group prediction that allows insurance companies to make a profit may be of only minor assistance to the clinician attempting to predict the behaviour of an individual patient.

## Actuarial predictions: learning the lessons of history

The principle underlying standardized risk assessment is simple. It began in the Canadian prison system, where administrators collected information about a large numbers of offenders, then collated it with reoffending data. Using simple statistics it was possible to construct statements of probability. If a prisoner had characteristics A and B, then the probability of reoffending was, say, 25%. If he had A and B combined with C, then that probability increased to 35%.

The life insurance industry uses the same method, and it is for that reason it is known as actuarial risk assessment. Insurance companies use mortality statistics to link deaths in a population with variables such as age, sex, and smoking. The associations are established by looking at history, the assumption being that deaths in the future will follow much the same broad pattern as in the past.

This reliance on history explains why insurers panicked when AIDS came along. Here was a new, significant cause of deaths in young people. Precisely because it was new it did not figure in any actuarial calculations, and the industry could have been bankrupted by a sudden increase in claims. The response was a reluctance to take on new business, combined with a general rise in premiums. The industry recognized large and incalculable risks associated with a new disease, so it acted conservatively or defensively. Only now, when history has provided actuarial data on AIDS, is it possible to calculate risk more accurately again.

History does not always repeat itself, but it almost repeats itself often enough to allow insurers to survive. When new diseases or cures enter the equation there are minor upheavals, then the maths are adjusted and it is business as usual. But what is good enough for the insurer may not be good enough for the clinician, and history is often a poor guide to the prediction of individual behaviour. It will be argued later that the proper place of historical or actuarial data is to inform a comprehensive assessment, not to substitute for it.

## Clinician or insurance salesman: individuals and groups

Insurers deal in group predictions, and the larger the group the more reliable the prediction. By the time we get down to the level of the individual patient—the smallest of all possible groups—there is little or no basis for accurate prediction. The best we can hope for is to make a statement of relative probability, conditional upon a range of circumstances.

One should be suspicious of any attempt to assign an absolute probability of violence to an individual. The most we can says is that an individual resembles a group or class of people in whom there is a specific probability of violent offending. For example, we know that the probability of non-sexual reoffending in convicted sex offenders is about 50% but we cannot say that an individual sex offender has a 50% probability of reoffending. The argument against such false logic was rehearsed above, in relation to ethnic origin and imprisonment. The same principles apply whenever we are tempted to assume that the characteristics of a group apply to an individual member of that group.

One of the themes running through this book is that not all errors are equal. Some are more serious than others, and it is a serious error for clinical services to treat an individual as nothing more than a typical representative of a group. At worst the error may amount to racism or another form of discrimination, and it conflicts with the emphasis of health services on respect for individual autonomy. Insurance companies can get away with this sort of behaviour, and I argue below that managers and planners are also permitted to operate on this lower moral plane, but clinicians need to be more careful.

## Other limitations: the lure of numbers

Actuarial risk assessment is in vogue at present. In part, this is a backlash against some pretty dubious practice in clinical risk assessment. Mental health professionals have been detaining patients on the basis of clinical risk assessments, with little systematic study of their decision-making. Research suggests that too many patients are detained for too long, at too high a level of security. A disproportionate number of these patients are women, members of an ethnic minority, or both, while the doctors signing the forms often belong to neither category. On the other hand, there is widespread concern about violence by the mentally ill, with doctors accused of being reluctant to detain patients until it is too late.

In this context, mental health services cannot afford the luxury of complacency about risk assessment. These problems have coincided with intense scrutiny and questioning, not to mention suspicion bordering on paranoia, directed at all professional elites. Politicians, and the people they represent, are no longer content to leave important decisions to the experts. They want to know how decisions are made, and they want to know how accurate those decisions are.

Actuarial measures of risk are bound to find favour in the fight for accountability and transparency. These scales make explicit the basis for judgements about risk, in a way that can be understood by judges, courts, tribunals, and the lay population. They may even express risk in a concrete, numerical manner. Some actuarial tests attach a percentage to the risk of offending over a given time period, rather than simply describing it as high or low. Leaving aside concerns about accuracy it is easy to understand the attractions of this approach, rather than relying on clinical opinion.

The use of percentages in this way is particularly seductive. Now we can use numbers like real scientists. Precise measurement is so much better than clinical intuition that it seems too good to be true and, following life's general rule, this rosy scenario is indeed too good to be true. The apparent certainty of the statistics masks serious problems. The flaws may not be serious enough to lead us to abandon the whole exercise, as some critics suggest, but they necessitate a health warning against unthinking use. As noted above, percentages derived from groups do not apply to an individual.

The search for scientific precision causes other problems, and they are best understood by looking at the example of the VRAG. The problems are common to all similar instruments but the VRAG is the most widely used example. Also, its authors invited criticism by claiming that actuarial methods should supplant clinical estimation of risk (Quinsey et al., 1998, p. 171). They argued that their scale was so superior to clinical methods that it should not be contaminated in any way by such judgements. The following section will show that a clinician would be reckless to follow their advice.

## The origin of the Violence Risk Appraisal Guide

The VRAG (Quinsey et al., 1998) was intended to be a pure, actuarial measure of risk, untainted by theory or clinical judgement. The authors studied 600 adult male patients released from a high security hospital in Ontario, Canada. Their outcome measure was violent reoffending and they collected a mass of data on each patient, using sophisticated statistical techniques to decide which of these items predicted a bad outcome.

The result was a list of 12 items weighted according to the strength of their statistical association with violence during the 7-year follow-up.

Total scores on the instrument have been divided into nine bins, along a spectrum of violence risk. Each bin has an attached probability of violence, expressed in percentage terms and relating to a seven-year time frame.

## Limitations of the Violence Risk Appraisal Guide

A critique of the scale begins with face validity. Even a glance at the items in Table 5.1 suggests some of them do not look right. Three of the four variables associated with reduced risk of violence do not make clinical sense. It is reasonable that an older patient presents a lower risk than a young one, but why should schizophrenia, serious injuries caused to the victim, or the fact the victim was a woman, provide any reassurance about future violence risk?

Defenders of the scale would argue that it does not need to make sense. The factors are derived from a statistical analysis of recidivism; they describe reality and should be accepted as facts. This would be a valid argument if we only wanted to apply the scale to the population on which it was created, that is, the original sample of patients discharged from the high security hospital at Penetanguishene in Canada. The VRAG allows a more or less accurate reconstruction of the historical events following their discharge. But clinicians are not historians. They are interested in different groups of patients, in different environments, in the here and now, and in the future.

The problems are illustrated by speculating about why these 12 items were found to be important. For most of them, the task is easy. There is a wealth of literature on the relationship between violence risk and psychopathy, conduct disorder and early childhood maladjustment. It would be surprising if any scale including these factors did not have some success in measuring violence risk.

Difficulties arise with the specific factors of schizophrenia, female victim, and extent of victim injury. The use of these factors as indicators of reduced risk is not consistent with the wider literature, so they may reflect specific

**Table 5.1** The 12 items of the Violence Risk Appraisal Guide (Quinsey et al., 1998)

| PCL-R Score | History of non-violent offending |
|---|---|
| Problems at junior school | Never married |
| Personality disorder | Schizophrenia (–) |
| Alcohol abuse | Extent of victim injury (–) |
| Separated from parents before age 16 | Age (–) |
| Failure on prior conditional release | Female victim (–) |

(–) after an item indicates a negative correlation with risk of violence.

features of the sample. What do we know about patients who were released from high security hospitals at that time?

Such patients can be divided broadly into the mentally ill, usually suffering from schizophrenia, and those with personality disorder. We know that, in general, the mentally ill present fewer problems of reoffending under supervision. Hence, the presence of schizophrenia indicates lower risk, but only in comparison with patients with personality disorder.

Another problem arises from the fact that the sample included only patients who were discharged. In patients with schizophrenia, fitness for discharge probably means that the symptoms are controlled by medication. Although the VRAG took no account of patients who were not discharged, it is reasonable to assume they included those whose mental illness did not respond to medication, or those who refused to comply with treatment. It is not surprising that treated patients with schizophrenia are less violent than patients with personality disorder, but it would be a serious mistake to draw any conclusions about untreated, or treatment resistant, patients with schizophrenia.

Turning now to victim gender and the extent of victim injury, we know also that many offenders with schizophrenia commit offences against close family members, typically mother or spouse. The offence is often driven by strong emotions that are specific to the victim. Removal of the victim, as in the case of matricide, in itself decreases the risk of recidivism. Hence, these offenders have a relatively low risk when properly treated and supervised.

The relative risk is distorted still further because psychopathic offenders who cause serious injury or death to female victims are often violent sexual predators who will find it difficult, if not impossible, to get out of a high security hospitals precisely because they are regarded as posing such a high risk of reoffending. As a result, they are likely to be under-represented in the sample of discharged patients on which the VRAG is based. Therefore, it is unreasonable to expect the VRAG to be of much use in assessing them. The VRAG sample included men who had caused serious injury to victims, or men whose victims were women, mainly when the offences had occurred in the course of schizophrenia. Men with psychopathic disorder who had committed these offences tended not to get into the sample because they were not discharged.

This speculation is supported by empirical evidence. Serial killers of women, who have already demonstrated their ability to offend repeatedly, may achieve low scores on the VRAG.

These are serious problems. In fact, they are serious enough to suggest that the VRAG should not be used for clinical purposes. The clinician does not want to be in the position of explaining to a court or tribunal why she has based her risk assessment on a scheme that attaches less future risk to the killing of women than to the killing of men. Similar concerns apply to explaining why schizophrenia should reduce the assessed violence risk, when the literature from general population studies shows that psychotic mental illness is associated with increased risk.

Defenders of the VRAG will point out that it has been validated in many populations, where it shows a reasonable correlation with violent recidivism. However, given its inclusion of psychopathy and other related items, it would be surprising if it showed no such correlation. The problem is that it achieves these positive results despite the inclusion of the items discussed above. VRAG loyalists look on these anomalies as minor quirks, the eccentricities of an elderly, lovable but dementing aunt.

The sentimental attachment is surely misplaced. The VRAG has served its purpose by helping to popularize actuarial risk assessment, but the time has come to pension it off so far as individual clinical assessment is concerned. If one is dealing with a group of patients who have already been judged fit for discharge from a high security hospital, the VRAG will do a reasonable job of estimating their risk of violent recidivism. It is not suitable for deciding whether or not a patient is ready for discharge.

Even when used in a limited role, there is one further qualification to be added. Actuarial instruments are expected to give reasonable results only if the world has remained substantially unchanged in the period since they were developed. Remember the problems caused to the life insurance industry by the arrival of AIDS, and the discussion above about history not repeating itself. The VRAG described a group of patients at a specific time and there is no reason to assume it would still give good results if the nature of the population changed as a result of variation in clinical practice.

## Summary: limitations of the VRAG

The VRAG is unfortunate in containing several items that lack face validity. Because it looks wrong, it is useful as an example but its fundamental problems apply to all actuarial instruments. These instruments rely on a description of a particular population at a point in time and assume the same description applies to other populations, at other times.

The VRAG suffers from having been devised on a special, select group of patients. The assumption that the original and present populations will behave in the same way is most likely to be valid if the original population was large and more or less identical to the population in which one is now applying the test. Another way of expressing this problem is to say that actuarial tests are on safe ground when taking a broad-brush approach to risk, using well-established, general risk factors. Again, we come back to previous offending, psychopathy and childhood pathology. These factors indicate a generally increased risk of recidivism, but specific predictions are likely to be misleading.

It is important to note that this is a problem of principle, not technique. The limitation is intrinsic to the actuarial method, no matter how well it is applied. If we attempt to make our description of a population more accurate in its detail, by using more sophisticated statistics or by gathering more information, it becomes less likely that the description will apply to a new population.

A good example is provided by morbid jealousy, which we know is often associated with violence. Most populations of mentally disordered offenders will contain men in whom morbid jealousy played a part in their violence, and it will appear as a risk factor for offending. If we constructed a detailed, sophisticated description of a group of mentally disordered offenders after follow-up, we could estimate how important morbid jealousy was in predicting violence in that group of men, but we could not expect that description to be accurate in detail for any other group. There would be a general tendency for morbid jealousy to be associated with violence, but we could not predict the strength of the association.

## Other actuarial methods and standardized assessments

Despite stating several times that it is presented mainly as an example of the limitations common to all actuarial instruments, it seems unfair to discuss only the VRAG in this section. Therefore I will mention briefly some other actuarial instruments.

### The Iterative Classification Tree (ICT, Monahan *et al.*, 2001)

The most sophisticated description of a mental health population is probably the ICT, developed by Monahan *et al.* (2001) as part of the Macarthur study of mental disorder and violence. Its claim to fame is that it uses a decision tree

**Table 5.2** The paradox of actuarial risk assessment

| |
| --- |
| 1. Actuarial instruments depend on a historical description of violence and its correlates in a particular population |
| 2. The more detailed and precise the description, the better it reveals correlates of violence |
| 3. History does not repeat itself |
| 4. The more detailed and precise the historical description, the less the findings will generalize to a new population or a new time |

rather than a simple list of variables associated with violence. The authors present statistics to show that this sequential approach provides a better description of violence risk in their study population, compared with a simple adding-up of risk factors.

The statistics may be persuasive, but the tree provides no escape from the paradox common to all actuarial studies. The ICT may be better history, but it is still history. By increasing the precision of the description of the original sample, we make it less likely that the findings will apply to new populations. This is psychiatry's equivalent of Heisenberg's uncertainty principle in physics; the more precise one element of a description, the less it is likely to apply in another setting. It is pointless to struggle against this inevitability by searching for ever more complex statistical descriptions. We need to accept the limitations of actuarial methods and look for new ways to use and supplement them in clinical practice.

Out of fairness to the VRAG it must also be emphasized that the ICT is at an earlier stage of development, so much so that when originally presented it had been tested only against the original, MacArthur study population. The process of developing an actuarial instrument involves first an accurate description of the original population, then testing of the pilot instrument on new populations. The VRAG has been extensively tested, whereas the ICT is still close to first base. Cooke (2000) has also pointed out that the ICT can only classify individuals as high or low risk and leaves some as uncertain or incapable of classification by this method—yet it is precisely the intermediate group with whom clinicians are most likely to need help.

### The Offender Group Reconviction Scale (OGRS) (Copas J and Marshall P, 1998)

OGRS has the great virtue of up-front honesty, by proclaiming itself a group instrument. It was developed by the Home Office (Taylor, 1999) for use with offenders serving community sentences in England and Wales, and its purpose was to predict the risk of all reoffending, not just violence. It has the other virtue of brevity, by using only five static factors: age, sex, number of previous convictions, number of custodial sentences while under 21 years of age, and seriousness of the index offence.

### The Level of Service Inventory—Revised (LSI-R, Andrews and Bonta, 1995)

This is an actuarial predictive scale using static (e.g. age, previous convictions) and dynamic factors (e.g. alcohol, accommodation problems). It predicts risk of reoffending rather than violence and also identifies need for probation supervision. As the name suggests, it was developed as a means of helping to estimate the level of supervision required by offenders. It is subject to all the

**Table 5.3** The 10 items of the Static 99 Actuarial Assessment (Hanson and Thornton, 2000)

| |
|---|
| 1. Young |
| 2. Ever lived with intimate partner |
| 3. Conviction for non-sexual violence at same time as index offence |
| 4. Previous convictions for non-sexual violence |
| 5. Previous sex offences |
| 6. Sentenced on 4 or more previous occasions |
| 7. Any convictions for non-contact sex offences |
| 8. Unrelated victims |
| 9. Stranger victims |
| 10. Male victims |

usual reservations about making decisions on individuals, but its potential value in service planning will be explored in a later section.

### Sex offender risk assessments

These include the Rapid Risk Assessment for Sex Offender Recidivism (RRASOR, Hanson 1997), The Sex Offender Risk Appraisal Guide (SORAG, Quinsey *et al.*, 1998), Static 99 (Hanson and Thornton, 2000—see Table 5.3), and Risk Matrix 2000. I could continue but this seems to be the correct point at which to say enough is enough.

How many actuarial instruments does a clinician need? Not that many, and none at all in many situations. Rather than carry on with a list, it is more relevant to consider how and when such scales can be useful in clinical practice. For those who want to read more there is plenty of relevant material in Cooke (2000), Cooke *et al.* (2001), and Kemshall (2002). The rationale and scoring method for the Static 99 are described in Harris *et al.* (2003).

Before considering the clinical application of standardized assessments, it is necessary first to digress into the topic of psychopathy and its measurement. The reason is simple. Psychopathy is fundamental to many standardized risk assessments, and it is impossible to understand these techniques without understanding psychopathy.

## Psychopathy

The term psychopathy is more or less synonymous with the categories of anti-social personality disorder (ASPD) in DSM IV and with dissocial personality disorder in ICD10. It has sometimes been referred to as sociopathy.

The range of different terms reflects the fact that this concept has been problematic throughout its long history. Pinel referred to it as 'manie sans delire', or a form of madness in which delusions, and other clear signs of mental illness, are absent. Without such signs, how can one make the diagnosis reliably? Where does ordinary criminality stop and psychopathy begin? As Maudsley (1874, p170) put it, this diagnosis 'has so much the look of vice or crime that many consider it an unfounded medical invention'.

Little progress was made over the following decades, as psychiatrists tried and failed to discard the diagnosis. For a long time, the only developments were changes in the name, in an (unsuccessful) attempt to shed pejorative and stigmatizing connotations. The underlying concept would not go away, but few people were comfortable with it. In part, the discomfort arose from diagnostic uncertainty. Was psychopathy just another word for criminality? The stalemate looked set to continue indefinitely, until Hare devised an operational definition, derived from Cleckley's concept of psychopathy.

## The Psychopathy Checklist

The Psychopathy Checklist, later to become the Psychopathy Checklist Revised (PCL-R), resurrected psychopathy as a useful clinical entity by allowing reliable diagnosis. Using this 20-item scale, it was possible to distinguish psychopathy from criminality. And once the condition was defined, it could be researched. There has been exponential growth of research using the PCL-R, well documented on Professor Hare's website (http://www.hare.org). In summary, scores on the PCL-R have been found to correlate with violence in samples drawn from a range of criminal justice and psychiatric populations.

The PCL-R gives a score from 0 to 40 as each of its 20 items is scored 0 (absent), 1 (probably or partially present), or 2 (definitely present). A screening version, the PCL-SV, has also been developed, using only 12 items to give a maximum score of 24. Both versions of the scale make use of case notes and an interview, and the PCL-R can be completed using case notes alone. This gives it an enormous advantage over other measures of personality. No matter how sophisticated, most such measures rely on self-report which is a serious problem because lying is a feature of psychopathy. Even if lying is not involved, self-report implies a degree of insight and self-reflection that is beyond the capacity of many patients. The PCL is unique in recognizing and measuring the tendency to deceive self and others.

## Psychopathy: diagnosis or dimension?

The presence of psychopathy is conventionally defined as a score of 30 or above in North America or, for various technical and social reasons, 25 or

**Table 5.4** The 20 items of the Psychopathy Checklist-Revised (PCL-R, Hare, 1991, pp. 73–77)

**Interpersonal/affective:**

1. Glibness/superficial charm
2. Grandiose sense of self-worth
3. Pathological lying
4. Conning/manipulative
5. Lack of remorse or guilt
6. Shallow affect
7. Callous/Lack of empathy
8. Failure to accept responsibility

**Social deviance:**

9. Need for stimulation/proneness to boredom
10. Parasitic lifestyle
11. Poor behavioural controls
12. Early behavioural problems
13. Lack of realistic long-term goals
14. Impulsivity
15. Irresponsibility
16. Juvenile delinquency
17. Revocation of conditional release

**Additional items:**

18. Promiscuous sexual behaviour
19. Many short-term marital relationships
20. Criminal versatility

above in Europe. It is important to remember, though, that all scales have a margin of error. It makes no psychometric sense, or any other kind of sense, to give the label psychopath to a man scoring 30, but not to a man scoring 28 or 29. Research demands that we draw the line somewhere, to allow comparisons between groups, but we should remember that this is a scientific device rather than a reflection of reality. In clinical situations there is a strong argument for thinking in terms of high, moderate, or low scores, rather than rigid categories.

The debate about the status of psychopathy continues. Should it be considered a personality characteristic, such as extraversion or neuroticism, of which an individual may have more or less? Or is it a diagnostic entity or

**Table 5.5** The 12 items of the PCL-SV (from Hart et al, 1995)

| |
|---|
| 1. Superficial |
| 2. Grandiose |
| 3. Deceitful |
| 4. Lacks remorse |
| 5. Lacks empathy |
| 6. Doesn't Accept Responsibility |
| 7. Impulsive |
| 8. Poor Behavioural Controls |
| 9. Lacks Goals |
| 10. Irresponsibility |
| 11. Adolescent Antisocial Behaviour |
| 12. Adult Antisocial Behaviour |

taxon, such as schizophrenia, in which case a patient has it or he does not? Hare's view is that there is a distinct disorder but this debate has little clinical relevance and soon gets bogged down in complicated statistics. In clinical practice a diagnosis is sometimes more convenient than a score but we need to remember there is a large margin of error, and any cut-off point is arbitrary.

In this context, it is encouraging to find that, in the MacArthur study of ordinary psychiatric patients in the USA, scores on the PCL-SV correlated with violence at levels below the usual cut-off for a diagnosis of psychopathy. The PCL score has clinical value, irrespective of whether or not diagnostic criteria are fulfilled. Note the stark contrast between psychopathy and a diagnostic entity such as schizophrenia. It is useful to know whether patients have a touch of psychopathy, whereas the idea of having a touch of schizophrenia is nonsensical. In other words, psychopathy is a useful concept even outside the group of serious offenders where it is most commonly found. A PCL score is a useful proxy measure of risk in any patient with a history of violence.

## The downside of psychopathy: labelling and stigmatization

We have seen that psychopathy can be reliably measured, even in offender populations where lying and deceit may be common. Scores on the PCL correlate with violence in populations of offenders and patients, even at levels below the point at which a diagnosis of psychopathy could be made. So what is the catch?

Problems arise mainly from the static nature of the measure. Most of the factors on the PCL are historical and they are scored on a lifetime basis, rather than present state: once a psychopath, always a psychopath. If one relies only on the PCL score, an offender may look as dangerous at the age of 90 as he did when he was 35. Intensive cognitive-behavioural treatment and community supervision may reduce the risk of violent or sexual recidivism by up to 50%, but it will leave the PCL score unchanged. Psychopathy can get you into trouble, but it cannot get you out. As it is not a measure of change it is of limited use when considering release or discharge.

These facts are bad enough in themselves, but there have also been suggestions that psychopaths are resistant to treatment, and that conventional interventions may even make them worse. Rice *et al.* 1992, this is a flawed study, mainly because the treatment involved would not be recognized today as a reasonable approach to reducing recidivism. It was very much of its time, the 1970s, and it included nude encounter groups alongside unstructured group therapies.

Other evidence is reviewed in D'Silva *et al* (2004). Conventional offending behaviour programmes within the UK prison system were associated with an increase in reoffending after discharge in prisoners with high PCL-R scores. One aspect of these findings that is often overlooked is that community supervision was effective in reducing reoffending, regardless of the level of psychopathy. It may be that we need to discard a conventional treatment model and think of psychopathy as a lifelong condition requiring rehabilitation and supervision to achieve and maintain a reduced risk of offending.

## Summary: psychopathy

The PCL is a reliable and valid measure of psychopathic personality and scores correlate with violence risk in many populations.

As the PCL score remains stable over time, it is useless as a measure of change. It is a useful baseline measure in any patient with a history of serious violence.

A high score on the PCL suggests that treatment may be more difficult and that the patient may not enter readily into a therapeutic alliance. Even so, long-term supervision is likely to reduce the risk of recidivism and there is no justification for excluding high scorers from services. Further information can be found in the review by Dolan and Doyle (2000).

The final part of this chapter is concerned with the place of actuarial assessment in clinical practice. It begins with a slight digression on the growth of the risk assessment industry, and its implications for the clinician.

## The violence risk assessment industry

The simple concepts underlying life insurance have led to the growth of the violence risk assessment industry, with a proliferation of different instruments. This is all very well for those inventing them, who can enjoy their 15 minutes of fame, but it is confusing for the clinician. When, if ever, is it necessary to use a standardized assessment? Which one should it be? What do I do when the results are worrying?

The answers to these and related questions depend on the context and the purpose of the assessment. How much is at stake? Is it a one-off assessment to inform a decision on release or discharge? Is it intended to guide treatment? Is it a measure of change? Choice in these different situations should be guided by three differences between instruments.

1. the quality of standardization

2. static versus dynamic variables

3. special features.

## The quality of standardization

There is an extensive literature on the factors associated with reoffending, so it is easy to choose items to include in a risk assessment instrument. The difficult part of this process is the standardization. Big numbers are needed, and the sample must be selected to allow for the possibility of bias resulting from age, sex, or ethnic differences. Most of the standardization has been done in Canada and the USA, and we cannot assume the same norms will apply in other countries, although initial results using the PCL-R in UK prison populations are encouraging.

Compared with the process of standardization, the content of the risk assessment instruments may be of less importance. In fact, when one looks at the range of actuarial measures in detail, there is a lot of cross-fertilization if not incest. The Static 99 turns out to be the bastard offspring of RRASOR and the SACJ (Hanson and Thornton, 2000). The same authors crop up again and again, designing the instruments, evaluating them then redesigning them. Within the scales the same items crop up again and again.

Unlike real incest this is all legal, not to say typical of academia, but clinicians are likely to feel excluded. Much of the debate in the literature (e.g. Kemshall, 2002, chapter 4) revolves around minor statistical differences that have no clinical relevance. Back in the real world, the key message is that actuarial instruments rely heavily on previous offending, conduct disorder and psychopathy, mixed up with evidence of sexual deviation or mental illness when relevant, then recycled or repackaged in various ways.

The differences between instruments are often differences in terminology or emphasis. Information may be coded in different ways, the weight given to specific items will vary, and some scales include specialized items, such as those relating to sex offending or mental illness, alongside the generic items relating to offending, psychopathy and childhood disturbance.

In many cases the borrowing of one scale from another is explicit. The VRAG (Harris *et al.*, 1993) and the Historical Clinical Risk-20 (HCR20, Webster *et al.*, 1997) both include a measure of psychopathy (the PCL-R or the shorter PCL-SV). The Violence Risk Scale (VRS, Wong and Gordon, 2000) also includes a measure of psychopathy.

The Sex Offender version of the VRS uses the Static 99 as an actuarial measure, and there is nothing wrong with this borrowing or inclusion of other scales. It is preferable to the practise of creating new scales for no good reason—there are more than 35 standardized measures of sexual offending risk in use in the USA, and it seems unlikely each can justify its claim to a niche, even in the world's marketing capital.

Risk scales have proliferated in recent years because it is easy to create new ones by adding items to the core features of offending, psychopathy, and childhood disturbance. The forces shaping this development are the same ones that created US supermarkets, their aisles stocked with 50 different cereals that are virtually indistinguishable from each other once you have got through the packaging. While a few people have made a lot of money from the risk business, the main motivation for developing new scales is the vanity of academics and their need to maintain production, which is just as pressing as the needs of cereal producers. But there are real disadvantages associated with a proliferation of new scales. The first one is a lack of standardization. New scales have to begin the process all over again, so some of them rely on small samples and are of unproven validity. Unless an existing scale has glaring problems, there must be a strong case for keeping it and improving standardization by using it on larger reference populations, rather than starting all over again. The whole point of the actuarial method is good standardization, and it makes no sense to abandon it in a fruitless search for the holy grail of a perfect measure. The attitude of the life insurance industry is that major change is needed only when a new disease comes along, and violence risk assessment should adopt a similar threshold for change.

A second major problem is that the proliferation of instruments leaves clinicians confused. Anyone who has visited a US supermarket will be familiar with the feeling of having too much choice and wanting one decent product without the need to wade through 49 rejects first. When it would take a lifetime to become familiar with all the possible options, it is tempting to abandon the whole enterprise and carry on with clinical assessment. The growing mountain of acronyms no longer serves the clinician and threatens to create a world in which nerds and techies argue the pros and cons of different instruments, having forgotten long ago that the aim of this process was to improve the clinical management of individual patients. There is an urgent need for simplification.

Standardization may also have different connotations for the clinician. As one aim of risk management is good communication, a scale becomes much more useful when it is used throughout a service and by different services. Agreement on a common standard may be more important than precisely which instrument is chosen, once we accept that the perfect actuarial instrument does not exist and will never exist.

When a clinician asks which instrument to use when assessing a sex offender, the correct answer most of the time will be that it does not make much difference in terms of the end result. The best advice is to choose a well-established instrument that is simple to administer and needs minimal training.

## Static versus dynamic variables

The hundreds of items used by all the different scales can be divided into two types: static or dynamic. Do they change, or do they stay the same? An example of a static factor is childhood conduct disorder, which is known to increase the probability of adult offending. While this historical factor is predictive, it will never change. It cannot be the target of treatment and it is useless as a guide to whether or not an offender's risk has reduced.

Dynamic factors are those such as substance misuse, intoxication, anger, or psychotic symptoms, all of which may change with time. Unlike static factors they are useful targets for treatment. We can measure change in dynamic risk factors as a guide to whether or not risk has been reduced. They may or may not be an accurate guide but that is a different question, and there is at least a theoretical possibility of using such measures to monitor progress.

In principle, we know that dynamic variables must be important in determining offending. After all, even the most dangerous offender is not offending for most of the time. It is reasonable to suppose that some change prompts the offence, whether it is intoxication, availability of a victim, or deterioration in mental state. As the clinician's role is to reduce the probability of violence, it is inevitable that most interest will be in dynamic variables. Some of the tension between general and forensic psychiatrists results from irritation that it is easy to use static factors to create a worrying risk assessment, when the real need is for help in reducing the risk by identifying and modifying dynamic factors.

The problem is that most actuarial risk assessments rely on static rather than dynamic factors. Examples include the VRAG and Sex Offender Risk

**Table 5.6** Clinician's guide to choosing an actuarial or standardized risk assessment

| Principle | Rationale |
|---|---|
| 1. Relevant to population under consideration | Pretty obvious. Scales designed on prisoners may not apply to patients and vice versa. Static measures cannot demonstrate change |
| 2. Relevant to risk concerned | Scales may be designed for general offending risk, violence risk, sexual or spousal assault, etc. The right answer is more likely to emerge from asking the right question |
| 3. Well established | The standardization is likely to be better. Also, as one of the aims is better communication, other clinicians are more likely to understand the findings if the scale is familiar. These considerations will generally outweigh any complex statistical differences in claimed accuracy |
| 4. Simplicity | Actuarial risk assessment depends on a small number of variables, so why complicate life? None of the scales can cope with individual variation, so save the complexity and idiosyncratic factors for your clinical assessment |
| 5. Minimal training | See 4. Life is too short, until it is clearly shown that complicated actuarial methods have advantages. Copyright may make some scales expensive without added benefit |
| 6. Good face validity | Standardization is meant to help transparency so you should be ready to explain your scores to patients, relations, courts or Tribunals. It is a good idea to avoid anything that seems to fly in the face of common sense or the scientific literature |

Appraisal Guide (SORAG), and the Static-99. The PCL-R, although a measure of personality rather than risk, is also a static measure.

It is not surprising that clinicians have reservations about the use of these instruments. If the clinical task is to reduce risk and rehabilitate patients, it is not helpful to be told that a patient is high risk, and that the characteristics making him so are permanent features of his case. There is a conflict of interest here, but it is between researcher and clinician rather than between general and forensic psychiatry. The researcher likes variables that are simple to measure and study in large populations, and static factors fit the bill. It is much easier to study the link between previous offending and recidivism, than to look at mental state or treatment. The clinician, on the other hand, wants to make the patient better, so his main interest is in things that can be changed.

In fact, the conflict of interest is apparent rather than real. Clinicians cannot afford to ignore static variables, which set the context in which they work. The best analogy is, again, gambling. The static, historical factors are a good guide to the size of the stakes in a particular case. If this goes wrong, will we be dealing with a death or with threats and shouting? The clinician who attempts to manage risk while ignoring the history throws the dice before knowing the stakes. That is how shirts are lost.

For their part, researchers need to produce data that are useful to clinicians. Just because something is difficult to study does not mean it cannot be studied. Although most of the research was done in non-clinical settings, there is a growing literature on dynamic risk factors for offending. The findings have supported the incorporation of dynamic variables in standardized measures of clinical risk, most notably the VRS (Wong and Gordon, 2000) and the HCR-20 (Webster *et al.*, 1995). Both include dynamic variables alongside more traditional static ones, such as a measure of psychopathy derived from the PCL-R. The VRS has only six static factors but 20 dynamic ones.

## Special features of risk assessment instruments

The main distinction is between tools that measure the risk of violent offending, and those that assess the risk of sexual offending. Although many sexual offenders have high psychopathy scores, others have low psychopathy and little tendency to offend apart from their sexual pathology.

Although there are many scales designed to assess recidivism in sex offenders, the common feature is a measure of deviant sexual orientation such as paedophilia. The risk of sexual recidivism is increased by a history of offences against strangers; by the inability to form enduring intimate relationships; by psychopathy; and by general criminality. The archetypal incest offender, who may commit repeated sexual offences over many years against children in his care, may present a low risk of sexual offending outside this context if the case is not accompanied by psychopathy.

It is important to note that risk does not equate to seriousness of offending, or to the extent of the damage caused to victims, or to the appropriateness of punishment. Sexual abuse within the family may inflict particular harm because it is repeated over a long period of time, involves a massive breach of trust, and interferes with normal emotional development—all in addition to the trauma that accompanies any sexual assault. For this reason, the courts tend to impose long sentences in the name of retribution and deterrence, and it is wrong in principle for mental health professionals to question this approach—as it is none of their business. The fact remains that the risk of sexual offending in other contexts is often low and may be best managed through childcare legislation, with the main aim being to prevent the offender from ever being in a position of power over children. By contrast, the risk is massively increased if the actuarial assessment shows the additional presence of offences against strangers, and deviant sexual interests in other contexts.

Some instruments address another form of domestic offending, namely spousal assault. They are based on the fact that the risk factors may be rather different from those that apply to violence outside the home.

An area of developing interest is in the assessment of recidivism risk in adolescent offenders. Following on from the work of Moffit (1993) it is possible to distinguish lifetime-persistent from childhood-limited delinquency, and we know that childhood characteristics often persist into adulthood. Lee Robbins showed that approximately 50% of children with a conduct disorder go on to develop personality disorder in adulthood. Equally, of course, the same study shows that 50% of such children do not go on to develop a personality disorder. Other studies have shown a correlation between temperament at age 3, and adult criminality (Stevenson and Goodman, 2001).

These indications of continuity between adolescence and adulthood suggest that it should be possible to develop standardized measures with predictive value, and an adolescent version of the Psychopathy Checklist has been developed.

The main practical issue is that the adolescent has had less time at risk in which to develop patterns of offending behaviour, making it more difficult to detect stable trends. The ethical problem is that we do not like to label young people, fearing that the label itself will do harm. Nevertheless, the developing body of evidence in favour of strong developmental continuities suggests that this argument may be outweighed by the desirability of early identification and intervention in cases at high risk of future problems.

## Standardized risk assessment in clinical practice

While enthusiasts argue that actuarial methods should supplant clinical estimation of risk (Quinsey *et al.*, 1998, p. 171), a more balanced review (Monahan *et al.*, 2001, pp. 129–136) concludes that the proper place of such instruments is as an adjunct to good clinical practice. The actuarial assessment acts as a backdrop or canvas, on which the real work of clinical risk management can begin. Note that the standardized assessments do not dictate any course of action but illustrate the issues around which the clinical decision must revolve. The low PCL-R score suggests that if the psychosis can be treated, the residual risk of violence will be low. A high PCL-R score, on the other hand, would have suggested a considerable ongoing risk of violence even after treatment of the psychotic

### Case Study

A 25-year-old student develops schizophrenia insidiously, over a period of about a year. Initial contacts with services are inconclusive and he has had no treatment when the illness becomes florid and he kills a close family member under the influence of delusions and hallucinations. It is accepted that there was no motivation for the offence, other than his psychotic symptoms. The court wishes to impose a hospital order but there is disagreement about whether he should go to medium or high security.

He has no previous convictions and grew up in a conventional family setting, with no behavioural problems during childhood. His PCL-R score is low (close to zero) and the VRAG, for all its imperfections, places him in a low-risk group.

symptoms, implying the need for more prolonged rehabilitation and treatment. In the present case, the decision on high versus medium security hinges on whether or not the psychosis can be treated safely in the less secure setting. A standardized assessment cannot provide the answer but it ensures that the right question is being asked.

## Mental illness versus personality disorder

In general, prediction from actuarial scales is easier in the case of personality disorder than in mental illness. In the Macarthur study of 1000 general psychiatry patients, psychopathy emerged as the best single predictor of violence (Monahan *et al.*, 2001, pp. 65–72). This is probably because of the relative stability of the traits that make up antisocial personality disorder or psychopathy.

Standardized assessments are useful in personality disorder assessment because clinical assessment is more uncertain in the absence of clear symptoms such as delusions and hallucinations. Actuarial measures help to ensure better selection and treatment of patients, and can keep therapy on track when there is a danger of drift, or losing sight of treatment objectives. The PCL-R, with its avoidance of self-report and reliance on records, has revolutionized the clinical assessment of antisocial personality disorder.

Once psychosis supervenes most bets, if not all, are off. Standardized assessments will identify the higher risk associated with co-morbid personality disorder or substance misuse, but they are disappointing in predicting violence in uncomplicated psychosis.

The absence of psychopathy is no guarantee that a psychotic person will not offend as a direct consequence of the psychosis. Anecdotal evidence suggests that there is an inherent unpredictability about psychotic violence that is not associated with co-morbidity. We know that a considerable proportion of new cases of schizophrenia present with violence (Humphreys *et al.*, 1992). There is no scope for prediction when the target event occurs before the diagnosis has become apparent.

None of this is an argument against using actuarial measures in psychosis but it is a reminder that they should only be used as part of a comprehensive clinical assessment. With the growth of the risk assessment industry, there are many anecdotal reports of risks not being taken seriously because the actuarial score was low, only for a delusion or a grudge against an individual to lead to a homicide.

## The problem of low base rates

As a general principle, prediction leads to more errors when the base rate of the event is low (Szmukler, 2003). Whatever method is used, if it is inaccurate there are bound to be more false positives in a population where the condition concerned is uncommon, so actuarial instruments give fewer false positives in populations where violence is frequent.

In fact, this is a good example of the tendency of statistical argument to obscure a simple point. If a blind man shoots fish in a barrel, he will have a better hit rate if there are more fish in the barrel. His shooting is just as inaccurate, whatever the number of fish.

The argument about low base rates has been used to argue that standardized violence risk assessments are more useful to the forensic psychiatrist than the general psychiatrist, and that even in forensic populations they may have unacceptably high error rates.

However, any method of risk assessment has more false positive errors when the baseline rate of violence is low, so the same reservations apply to unstructured clinical assessment in such populations. The converse argument is that the clinician working in an environment where violence is relatively rare is in most need of help in identifying higher risk patients. The forensic psychiatrist can safely assume that all his patients present a risk, whereas the general psychiatrist would make the opposite assumption and gain most from a simple screening test to indicate patients who are more worrying.

The statistical argument about base rates is a distraction. The true issue is one of cost benefit: the use of such instruments has a cost in manpower, training, and time, and their use may not yield sufficient benefits in populations where violence is uncommon.

## Planners, managers, and auditors

I have already mentioned the different moral imperatives and obligations that apply to people in these groups, as compared with clinicians. Like insurers they are concerned with groups of people, so the arrival of actuarial risk assessments really does mean birthdays and Christmas all at the same time. There is no longer an obligation to agree without question to the demands of forensic services for extra resources simply because they deal with dangerous patients. Tough questions are now easy to ask. How dangerous are your patients, compared with patients in other services or other areas?

It is not that simple, of course—but it is almost that simple. There is bound to be a bit of variation, but if patients in a high secure or high dependency service are not scoring higher on standardized measures of violence risk, there is every reason to ask difficult questions. There may well be good answers, but the dialogue is necessary and good for patients.

The need for caution relates, as usual, to individuals. Standardized methods provide no better results for individuals when interpreted by a manager than when interpreted by a clinician. The larger the group, the more useful these instruments are likely to be. I look forward to the comparison of UK forensic

**Table 5.7** The place of standardized measures of risk in clinical practice

| Clinical situation | Role of standardized assessment |
| --- | --- |
| General mental health setting, no clinical pointers to violence risk | No advantages unless there are specific indications<br>May be helpful in audit or service planning, as in any setting |
| General mental health setting, patient has history of violence or other clinical pointers to violence risk | PCL-SV?<br>HCR20? (see next chapter)<br>In psychotic patients, the first priorities are good assessment of mental state and assertive treatment of the mental illness |
| General mental health setting, patient with history of serious violence | PCL-SV and any standard measure of violence risk (or HCR20) offers advantages over clinical methods alone<br>Consider forensic opinion |
| Forensic mental health service | PCL-SV or PCL-R, and any standard measure of violence risk (or HCR20) offer significant advantages over clinical methods alone |
| Sex offender assessment for civil or criminal court | Static 99 or similar helpful/essential<br>PCL-SV helpful/essential |
| Personality disorder services | PCL-SV or PCL-R virtually essential for offenders<br>Standardized measure of violence risk also virtually essential in those with a violence history<br>Standardized, dynamic measures are likely to improve treatment |

units to those in the rest of Europe and across the Atlantic. Actuarial measures of risk plotted against staffing levels and per capita costs would be a good place to start.

## Summary: standardized assessment for the clinician

Standardized measures are ideal for planners and managers but the advantages for clinicians are more circumscribed. Unthinking use to replace clinical assessment will lead to serious errors and is indefensible, but careful use can enhance clinical assessment. In some clinical situations, the use of actuarial measures offers such big advantages that they are virtually mandatory. Table 5.7 summarizes some of these situations.

One of the most important conclusions of this chapter is that standardized methods are no substitute for clinical practice but can enhance it. The next chapter will consider attempts to combine standardized and clinical methods in a systematic way.

## Chapter 6

# Structured clinical assessment of violence risk: The thinking man's approach

## Introduction

The previous chapter showed that standardized risk assessment is not a substitute for clinical assessment. The search for better scales will not solve all the problems of the actuarial approach, because some are inherent to the method. It is good enough for the insurance industry or the service planner, dealing with large and anonymous populations, but it is not good enough for the clinician working with individuals.

While standardized methods cannot replace clinical skills, they can improve them. In an ideal world, clinicians would use actuarial data to inform a clinical assessment tailored to the individual patient and his or her circumstances. Static, background risk factors can be combined with dynamic risk factors relating to the patient's present state, and the clinical assessment should take account of any quirks or idiosyncrasies that affect violence risk. The output will not be a percentage measure of risk, which is never accurate, but a risk management plan. A comprehensive risk management plan describes the risks in detail, estimates their magnitude and imminence, identifies factors that increase or decrease the risk, then sets out actions for managing those risks. Not all risks will be of equal importance, so the final step is to prioritize parts of the action plan.

The combination of standardized and clinical methods is known as the structured clinical assessment of violence risk (SCAVR). The rest of this chapter describes it in more detail and, as in the previous chapter, a specific instrument is used to illustrate the general principles. For SCAVR the chosen instrument is the HCR20 (Historical Clinical Risk-20; Webster *et al.*, 1997), which is widely used on both sides of the Atlantic.

**Table 6.1** The Structured Clinical Assessment of Violence Risk (SCAVR)

| |
|---|
| Step 1: Collection of data from records, patient interview and informants |
| Step 2: Standardized assessment of static and dynamic risk factors |
| Step 3: Consideration of idiosyncratic risk factors |
| Step 4: Description of violence risks, including nature, likely victims, and factors increasing and decreasing the risk |
| Step 5: Description of plans to address the risks, including contingency plans |
| Step 6: Assign priorities |

I should declare my prejudices at the outset by stating that the HCR20 is my preferred method of violence risk assessment, partly because it is the one I know best. And I am not alone in my preference for it. The HCR20 is widely used in Canada, and several forensic services in the UK have adopted it as a routine measure. My favouritism has limits, and I should emphasize that most of the following comments would apply equally well to any system of structured clinical assessment of violence risk.

I suspect that the HCR20, and other methods of SCAVR, have become popular because they help clinicians without telling them what to do. Structure is present because the team is obliged to collect and consider specified information before making plans, but the clinical team makes the final decisions. Choices are informed but not constrained by information collected systematically.

Others see this strength of the HCR20 as a weakness. Some clinicians are disappointed that the decisions and judgements remain with them; you have to fill in a lot of extra forms, but you still have to make tough choices at the end of the process. If this seems like extra work for little extra reward, the fault lies with the false promises of actuarial methods. They tempted us with a vision of a world in which we just tick the boxes and an infallible computer tells us the right answer. However, we know life is not really like that, and clinical practice consists of making choices in a complex situation where there are no right answers. By way of consolation, it is the uncertainties that make clinical work interesting and demanding. If actuarial methods held all the answers we would soon be replaced by robots. Until that day, a structured clinical approach can help us to do the job better.

The critical observer may also protest that SCAVR goes beyond assessment into risk management, but this is an advantage rather than a defect. Violence is not neutral. It is always a bad result. Good assessment therefore implies management aimed at improving the outcome.

# The HCR-20: risk assessment becomes risk management

The HCR20 begins by specifying information that must be collected in three domains: Historical (10 items), Clinical (five items), and Risk Management (five items). The items are listed in Table 6.2.

Each of these 20 items can be scored as definitely present (2), probably or partially present (1), or absent (0). The definitions for each item are included in Webster *et al.* (1997), and they are a major part of training in the use of the HCR20. They are not intended to be operational but require judgement and the exercise of discretion by the rater. In order to illustrate this point, an example of an item definition appears in Table 6.3.

**Table 6.2** The 20 items of the HCR20 (Webster *et al.*, 1997)

**Historical items**

| |
|---|
| H1: Previous Violence |
| H2: Young Age at First Violent Incident |
| H3: Relationship Instability |
| H4: Employment Problems |
| H5: Substance Use Problems |
| H6: Major Mental Illness |
| H7: Psychopathy |
| H8: Early Maladjustment |
| H9: Personality Disorder |
| H10: Prior Supervision Failure |

**Clinical items**

| |
|---|
| C1: Lack of Insight |
| C2: Negative Attitudes |
| C3: Active Symptoms of Major Mental Illness |
| C4: Impulsivity |
| C5: Unresponsive to Treatment |

**Risk management items**

| |
|---|
| R1: Plans Lack Feasibility |
| R2: Exposure to Destabilizers |
| R3: Lack of Personal Support |
| R4: Non-compliance with Remediation Attempts |
| R5: Stress |

**Table 6.3** Definition of 'Item C1. Lack of Insight' in the HCR20 (Douglas *et al.*, 1973, pp. 50–51)

| 0 | No lack of insight |
|---|---|
| 1 | Possible/less serious lack of insight |
| 2 | Definite/serious lack of insight |

This item refers to the degree to which the assessee fails to acknowledge and comprehend his or her mental disorder, and its effect on others. Such lack of insight can be expressed in many forms. Some persons with clearly evident major mental illnesses are unable or unwilling to see that they will likely act violently without regular use of prescribed medication. Others have difficulty realizing the importance that a well-structured support group may have in averting violence. Yet others have little comprehension of their generally high levels of anger and dangerousness.

The sample definition in Table 6.3 illustrates several points. It is not an operational measure. It does not specify precisely how to arrive at a particular rating. Instead it gives examples of how a lack of insight may manifest itself. The clinician has discretion over the extent to which a particular patient's behaviour is consistent with the example, so it follows that only experienced clinicians should use the measure. Instruments like the HCR20 are not an alternative to proper clinical training.

Although clinicians require specific training to use the HCR20, its relevance to ordinary practice is obvious from the item definition. Lack of insight is not an obscure feature of the patient, to be measured only in order to complete a scale. It is core clinical material. If you do not know the level of your patient's insight, you cannot manage the violence risk. The same goes for compliance and many of the other items. Given the basic training in its use, a clinician with knowledge of the patient will find it easy to complete the HCR20 because most of the ratings concern things he or she knows already. The only exception is psychopathy, Item H7, which is rated using the PCL-SV (see Chapter 5). The PCL-SV has its own specific training requirements but it is also easy to complete for any clinician familiar with the patient.

Because the items of the HCR20 rely on example and clinical judgement rather than operational definitions, they are not intended to reach the level of precision in scoring that is associated with psychometric tests such as the Wechsler Adult Intelligence Scale (WAIS see Chapter 5). The nature and purpose of these two scales is completely different, and the HCR20 only makes sense when integrated into clinical practice. Both the HCR20 and the WAIS can help the clinician but, unlike the WAIS, the HCR20 also requires the clinician's input and is useless without it. The point of the HCR20 is to use it to formulate a good risk management plan, rather than to arrive at an accurate score. In fact, I argue later that the score is of little value and it is better simply to consider whether items are present or absent.

Clinicians also like the HCR20 because the items were chosen for their known association with violence risk. As it is based on the scientific literature there are no counter-intuitive items like those found in the VRAG (where, for example, schizophrenia reduces the estimated risk of violence—see Chapter 5). The HCR20 makes clinical sense and has good face validity.

## The HCR20 and prediction

In broad terms, the *H*istorical, *C*linical, and *R*isk management) groups relate to past, present, and future. The Historical items are concerned with past behaviour, personality and mental illness. The Clinical items relate to current mental state and behaviour, and the Risk Management items relate to predicted functioning in the future. The latter items include the feasibility of future plans; the likely presence of stressors and destabilizers in the patient's environment; the presence or absence of personal support; and the likelihood of compliance with treatment. Although these items relate to the future and are therefore true predictions, they are not predictions that require a crystal ball. It is fairly easy to make such estimates in a patient who is well known to services, and these items have a high degree of inter-rater reliability.

The problems associated with prediction were discussed in a previous chapter. While accepting that we cannot foretell the future, any attempt at risk management has to be based on educated guesses about how the future may look. For example, Item R1 'Plans Lack Feasibility' refers to the need for an agreed, realistic care plan. It seems reasonable to consider problems in this area when considering risk, and it is possible to rate this item reliably, even though it relates to the future.

As an illustration of the value of this exercise, consider three points arising from the Ritchie report on Clunis (Ritchie *et al.*, 1994). First, any clinician reading the report is likely to conclude that the discharge plans were unlikely to succeed. Although stable at the point of discharge, it was predictable the patient would soon be homeless, without support, non-compliant and psychotic. In other words, it is possible to achieve a high level of inter-rater reliability even when considering something as nebulous as future behaviour.

Second, the Clunis case shows how important it is to consider the future, and how bad practice can get when clinicians attempt to ignore it. Assuming they acted in good faith, the professionals involved can only have discharged Clunis by concentrating on his mental state at the time while avoiding any thought of how he may look shortly afterwards. The structured clinical assessment of violence risk may not be a panacea, but it is a vast improvement on what was done in this case.

The third point is that the Ritchie report led the UK Government to introduce the Care Programme Approach (CPA), which is based on planning for the future and includes regular reviews. The HCR20's inclusion of items oriented towards the future means it fits easily into the CPA framework, as would any type of structured clinical assessment of violence risk.

## Scoring or rating in structured clinical assessment of violence risk

As noted above, the standard items of the HCR20 can each be rated absent (0), partially or probably present (1), or definitely present (2). The obvious next move is to add them together, to give a possible range of 0–40. Avoid the obvious. The whole point of SCAVR is that it is not an actuarial measure of risk, and once the risk assessment is reduced to a number it is hard to avoid thinking of it in actuarial terms. In fact, I regard this as one of the main sources of error in applying the HCR20.

Once a patient is reduced to a number, we assume that a 15 is higher risk than a 10, and a 25 higher than a 20. That may be so or it may not, and the rank ordering of cases according to HCR20 scores is misleading. Sometimes only a few items are positive but a single feature, such as a monosymptomatic delusion, may produce a high risk of serious violence. For this reason the exercise of clinical discretion is mandatory, and one should never allow a preoccupation with scores and numbers to lead to neglect of the clinical assessment.

Despite these reservations, the numbers cannot be dismissed entirely. A better way of using them is to consider the number of items rated 1 or 2, i.e. probably or definitely present. Clinicians using the scale soon get an impression of what is usual in their service, so the assessment draws attention to cases that are out of the ordinary. For example an acute, intensive care ward will often have patients with four or five Clinical items present. Many of them will also have four or five Risk Management items present. As a result the C and R items are not so useful in discriminating between cases, and variation in the number of Historical items may be a better indicator of differences.

I develop this approach in the next chapter, when applying the HCR20 retrospectively to patients who have killed. The study assumes that teams ought to give priority to patients who have most or all risk factors in all three categories, and this is probably a reasonable assumption. Even in these extreme cases, it is important to note that the presence of risk factors does not dictate any particular course of action except, perhaps, the formulation of a risk management plan.

## Description of violence risks

The totting up of risk factors is not a risk assessment. It is the preliminary work that lays the ground for a comprehensive risk management plan. That risk management plan has three steps as shown in Table 6.4. You should know the risk factors before addressing these questions but the risk factors do not provide the answers. Also, the questions have to be addressed even if some of the risk factors are unknown. It is here that clinical judgment comes in and takes over the process.

The three steps are:

i. Description of feared scenarios of violence

ii. Development of a risk management strategy

iii. Prioritisation of the case and arrangements for review

Table 6.4 presents the framework for an ideal, comprehensive risk assessment. It is a world away from simplistic notions of risk as high or low, or attempts to portray risk as a number or score. It is qualitative and relative rather than absolute. It does not attempt to specify the precise level of risk but it tells you what will increase or decrease it. It is also based on the assumption that risk assessment is pointless without risk management.

Table 6.4 encompasses an enormous amount of information and I shall now expand upon the work involved in each step.

*Step i. Description of feared scenarios of violence*

The feared scenarios are an opportunity for the team to assume the worst and to set out their worries on paper. What could go wrong? A patient may have more than one feared scenario. For example, it is common to find patients who present a risk of serious violence when in the community without medication, and under the influence of illicit drugs. The same patient may also present a risk within hospital of minor assaults on staff or other patients, irrespective of whether he is medicated or intoxicated. The factors contributing to the risks of different types of violence may not be the same, so the management strategies would be different. In this simplistic case detention in hospital may control the risk of serious violence in the community but it would increase the risk of minor assaults in hospital, which require another management strategy.

Although each scenario may have different risk factors and its own risk management strategy, the process does not go on for ever. In practice most patients have no more than two or three feared scenarios of violence and many have only one. Also, the same scenarios recur again and again in clinical practice.

**Table 6.4** Detailed description of violence risks and management (after Webster et al, 1997)

| Step 1: describe likely scenario | Step 2: develop management strategy | Step 3: determine priority |
|---|---|---|
| **Nature**<br>♦ What kinds of violence might this person commit?<br>♦ Who are the likely victims?<br>♦ What is the likely motivation? | **Risk factors**<br>♦ What events or circumstances might increase or decrease the patient's violence risk? | **Priority**<br>♦ What level of effort or intervention will it take to prevent this person from committing violence? |
| **Severity**<br>♦ What would be the harm (physical or psychological) to victims?<br>♦ Is it likely the violence might escalate to life-threatening levels? | **Monitoring required**<br>♦ How can we monitor warning signs?<br>♦ What events or circumstances should trigger a re-assessment? | **Immediate action**<br>♦ What steps should be taken immediately to prevent violence? |
| **Imminence**<br>♦ How soon might the violence occur?<br>♦ Are warning signs to suggest the violence risk is increasing or imminent? | **Treatment**<br>♦ What treatment (biological, social or psychological) could help to reduce the violence risk? | **Case review**<br>♦ When should the case be scheduled for routine review?<br>♦ What should trigger early review? |
| **Frequency/duration**<br>♦ How often might the violence occur — once, several times, frequently?<br>♦ Is the violence risk chronic or acute (i.e., time-limited)? | **Supervision**<br>♦ What supervision or surveillance could be used to manage this patient's violence risk? | |
| **Likelihood**<br>♦ In general, how frequent or common is this type of violence?<br>♦ How frequently has this person committed this type of violence?<br>♦ How likely is it that this person will commit this type of violence? | **Victim safety planning**<br>♦ What steps can be taken to protect likely victims? | |

Other than the need for some evidence in support, there are few rules for generating scenarios. Usually they are based on what the patient has done in the past. It seems sensible to include possible repetition of whatever violence has gone before. If there have been threats, an obvious scenario involves the patient carrying out the threats. The aim at the outset is to think the worst and to be over-inclusive. It is better to consider a risk then decide it needs no particular action, than not to consider it at all.

Some of the questions look impossible. How can we know future motivation for violence? How can we guess the identity of likely victims? Sometimes these questions are impossible, but in other cases they are easy and the solution lies in the past. If we know how and why a patient was violent in the past, we begin with the possibility that a similar scenario will be re-enacted in the future. Once we adopt this approach Table 6.4 begins to look like common sense. If a team is managing violence risk in the present, they need to look at what has happened in the past and plan for the possibility that it will happen again.

Of course, the past is never an exact replica of the future; life is full of surprises and not all of them are pleasant. We cannot plan for all contingencies but the approach outlined here ensures we address the obvious ones – which brings us back to one of the themes of this book, that not all violent acts are equal.

A patient will occasionally commit a violent act out of the blue, out of character for him, and with no warning. C'est la guerre, as French psychiatrists presumably say when things go badly and unexpectedly wrong. And a subsequent inquiry ought to say the same, if at much greater length and expense; it is unreasonable to criticize a service when care was reasonable and violence unforeseen. Scenario-planning could not have helped much because the warning signs were not there to be found. But the situation is quite different when the act of violence is more of the same, or just the latest and most serious in a series of similar acts. Clinicians will then be judged harshly for having failed to take account of an obvious risk, and scenario-planning would have revealed some of those risks. In other words scenario-planning gives most emphasis to the type of violence we can least afford to miss-and that is a good thing.

*Step ii. Development of a risk management strategy*

Whilst in theory the number of violence scenarios is infinite, in practice the same few situations recur with monotonous and depressing regularity. A non-compliant patient relapses, takes drugs then assaults family member/friend/fellow resident of hostel. A male patient assaults his partner when he is unwell, because of his jealousy and/or her infidelity. Themes of non-compliance, relapse and intoxication occur again and again, with many variations around the edges.

Frequent warning signs in the mentally ill include relapse and non-compliance, from which case management strategies follow automatically. Victim safety planning is often forgotten even though we know that relations and carers are disproportionately likely to be the victims of violence by the mentally ill. Protective factors tend also to be neglected but they should be part of any risk management plan.

*Step iii. Prioritisation of the case and arrangements for review*

The final step acknowledges that we live in the real world, where there are competing demands for time and attention. There is little room for absolutes. The only mandatory requirements are that decisions should be taken with eyes open to the possible consequences; actions should be defensible in terms of prevailing professional standards; and they should be justified in writing. The whole point of defensible practice is that it can be defended, and the essence of risk management is setting out one's defence in advance.

The principle is open to caricature as an attempt to get one's retaliation in first. Certainly, if we take the principle too far we enter the realms of defensive practice but there is plenty of room for sensible safety measures before that point is reached. The treatment of mental illness involves a large measure of unpredictability; transparent, documented decisions about the priority given to a case offer protection to staff on the rare occasions when things go seriously wrong.

There is a predictive element to the structured clinical assessment of violence risk but it develops from knowledge of a patient's actual or threatened violence in the past. The ability to incorporate idiosyncratic features of a case is crucial, and it is easy to make mistakes if this aspect is forgotten. The better the team knows the patient, the easier it should be to do the risk assessment. The HCR20 is not an actuarial instrument and it is meant to support and inform clinical judgment, rather than to replace it. It is in direct contrast to simplistic and misleading attempts to reduce risks to numbers.

## The case against SCAVR

Three main criticisms of SCAVR warrant further discussion. The first is that the method is nothing new and leaves the team to make the difficult decisions. Like all the best criticisms this one has a strong element of truth. SCAVR is little different from the best clinical assessments of risk because good clinicians impose their own structures. Unfortunately, most clinical assessments do not achieve the standards of the best. Facts are overlooked. Likely scenarios are not considered. The value of the structured clinical approach is that it helps to raise all assessments to the standards we achieve when working at our best.

It is also true that SCAVR leaves the difficult judgments to the clinicians, but this is a strength rather than a weakness. Management of violence risk is difficult because there are few certainties and no definitive right answers. There is a constant balancing of the rights of the individual patient against the rights of others. We can never know the future so we never know whether decisions are right or wrong until it is too late. With all this uncertainty, it is not surprising that clinicians grasp for tests, scales and numbers that will take the tough decisions for them. But they are grasping at an illusion. However elaborate the standardized assessment, in the end it leaves the clinician with a difficult decision. That is what clinicians are paid for. Many will respond that they are not paid enough, but at least we can console ourselves with the knowledge that machines will not be replacing us for some time yet.

The second criticism is that structured clinical assessment is a lot of trouble and not worth the time or effort. I deal more fully with the problem of resources in a later chapter. There is always a balance to be struck between costs and benefits. In a patient with no history of violence and no obvious indicators it may not be worth undertaking the process (although it is usually quick to complete in such patients as there are so many obvious negatives). In patients with a history of serious violence – and I include in that category anyone with a criminal conviction for violence, a history of using weapons, unprovoked assaults, assaults on strangers or sexual assaults – the balance of risks favours a full violence risk assessment. And a full violence risk assessment ought to address the questions in table 6.4. There is no short cut. If you have not attempted to answer these questions you have not done a comprehensive risk assessment.

Again we return to clinical judgment. A clinician has to weigh up what is known of the risks and decide when it is worth undertaking a full assessment. The mistake is to assume you can know the risks without doing the assessment.

A third criticism is that SCAVR may be good at identifying risks but it is pointless because there is nothing the team can do to change them, whether because of lack of resources; the constraints of the law; or the unwillingness of patients to follow advice. This is the ostrich position, preferred by those who are comfortable with head in sand and fingers crossed. It may serve clinicians reasonably well throughout an entire career because the risks of violence in mental illness are not so great. One can easily reach retirement before a disaster happens. But it is a form of gambling and most clinicians prefer not to take unnecessary risks, particularly when the stakes are so high.

Worse still, the ostrich position is disastrous for service development. If we abandon assessment out of fear of what we will uncover, we never identify deficiencies in services and we never deal with them. Patients continue to receive a service that is not as good as it could be, and we hand on the deficiencies to those who come after us. The sadness and futility of this approach to life is self-evident.

## Violence risk assessment in special groups

Many people turning to this section will be disappointed that it is so short. Violence risk assessment is often seen as more complicated than it is, with the expectation that different groups of patients will have different risk factors for violence, with a different set of rules that have to be learned if it is to be done correctly. The truth is that violence risk management in any group of patients assumes a high standard of clinical care, which requires the appropriate knowledge and skills, but the principles of risk management are pretty much the same for any group of patients. So if you know how to look after patients with learning difficulties and you have a general framework for structured clinical assessment of violence risk, the next step is to get on with it. There is little to be gained by waiting for specific instruction in risk management in a particular group, with the possible exception of adolescents.

The underlying factors determining violence risk have been well rehearsed in previous chapters and include: previous violence; mental disorder; psychopathy; childhood disruption and delinquency; early onset of problems; non-compliance; lack of response to treatment; substance misuse; unrealistic plans; lack of support; impulsivity; irritability; and stress. In general terms, each of these features is likely to be associated with violence risk, whatever the diagnosis or demographic characteristics. If you are called on to manage violence risk in the only known case of Furtwangler's syndrome, manifested in a Transylvanian hermaphrodite, you will still want to know the extent of previous violence and whether they had a bad childhood, plus all the other factors mentioned above, before you start to consider the idiosyncratic features.

The value of specialist skills and experience is that they allow better measurement of the risk factors for violence, and better management of identified needs, but the underlying factors are generally the same.

### General psychiatry

OK, so it is not a specialist area but it deserves mention because it has been slower than forensic psychiatry in embracing risk assessment, for obvious reasons, and because some parts of it still hold out against the principle. Most mentally ill homicides occur in general psychiatry, because that is where most of the patients are treated. General psychiatry has a desperate need for good violence risk management but resources are tight.

Not every patient can have a full violence risk assessment but it is probably reasonable to suggest that patients with severe mental illness and a history of violence should receive a fuller assessment. The state-of-the-art in this respect is structured clinical assessment of violence risk, so that is what has to be recommended. That may not be possible but the reasons for not doing it should be stated. All services should have access to HCR20 or similar, and once there is access there can be a waiting list and protocols for prioritization of cases.

If people want to argue with this suggestion, the argument should not be with me. I would guess that carers and commissioners expect psychotic patients with a history of violence to have a full violence risk assessment, so any argument should be with them.

Relationships with forensic services are sometimes difficult but general services should make more use of them, if only as second opinions. If a SCAVR comes up with worrying results, the next step should be a referral to forensic services for advice. Structured risk assessment tools provide a good basis for agreement on the relationship between forensic and general services, and may help to resolve awkward disputes about where a patient belongs.

Many general psychiatrists regard forensic opinions as unrealistic in recommending levels of treatment or supervision that are unattainable in practice. I understand the complaint but would defend the principle that it is correct to say what a patient needs and then to consider what can be provided in the real world as a secondary question. There is nothing wrong with recommending something that cannot be provided, nor is there anything wrong with not providing it, so long as the reasons are valid and well documented.

Finally, lest this all gets too complicated, the risk management priority for most general services should be an assertive treatment policy and effective policies and procedures for detecting and responding quickly to non-compliance with medication. A service in which all patients with serious mental illness and a history of violence take their prescribed medication has the luxury of time and space to think about more refined aspects of its violence risk management policies.

## Adolescents

It goes without saying that the family will often be of much greater importance in an adolescent, necessitating a wider assessment. This is a general feature of adolescent mental health and will not be considered in detail here. Turning to the specifics of risk assessment, there are two main problems complicating the process in young people. First, the peak age for delinquency is between 15 and 17 years. In terms of signal detection theory there is a lot of noise in the system. How does one distinguish ordinary delinquency from more sinister forms, without unnecessarily stigmatizing young people? We are slow to use diagnostic labels because they may do more harm than good, so we need strong evidence before attaching the label of high violence risk.

The second problem is the lack of history in a young person. Patients in their thirties have had time to build up a track record on which to base an assessment, whereas many 15 year olds have not. Greater uncertainty is inevitable.

There is no complete solution to these problems, but considerable progress has been made in recent years. Moffitt (1993) made a distinction between adolescence-limited and life-course-persistent delinquency, with the latter predictive of personality disorder and offending in adulthood. The life-course-persistent delinquent tends to have deep-seated problems with personal relationships, whereas the adolescence-limited delinquent frequently has good relationships with (often equally delinquent) peers. It seems certain that there will be a degree of continuity with adult psychopathy, and any assessment of a delinquent adolescent should include an attempt to place him on this spectrum.

Forth *et al.* (2003) published Hare's Psychopathy Checklist-Youth Version, intended for use in male or female offenders between the ages of 12 and 18. Like the PCL-R it has 20 items, as follows: 'impression management; grandiose sense of self worth; stimulation seeking; pathological lying; manipulation for personal gain; lack of remorse; shallow affect; callous/lack of empathy; parasitic orientation; poor anger control; impersonal sexual behavior; early behavior problems; lacks goals; impulsivity; irresponsibility; failure to accept responsibility; unstable interpersonal relationships; serious criminal behavior; serious violations of conditional release; and criminal versatility'.

It is to early to say how successfully the scale has overcome the practical problems involved in the assessment. There is also the more difficult question of how the scale will be used or misused, and I would have grave anxieties about its use for decision-making purposes outside the context of a full clinical assessment. However good the assessment technology, there must be more potential for change in a 13 year old than in a 30 year old, which means that any attempt at prediction should be accompanied by an even larger pinch of salt than usual. Those who wish to follow the evolving story are referred to Robert Hare's website, http://www.hare.org, which maintains an updated list of references.

There is now a Structured Assessment of Violence Risk in Youth (SAVRY, Borum *et al.*, 2002), which is closely modelled on the HCR20 approach. The SAVRY has been widely adopted by adolescent forensic mental health services in the UK.

## Women

There are many statistical differences between male and female offenders but it is useful to remember that, within biological constraints, women can do most things male offenders can do but they choose to do them less often. In other words there are fewer predatory female offenders than male but they exist and, as individuals, present as much of a risk as the commoner male equivalent.

The principles of SCAVR are the same as in men, and factors that indicate increased risk in men are likely to indicate the same in women. Potential problems concern the extent to which gender may affect the measurement of characteristics. Impulsivity, for example, may manifest itself differently in women than in men, which could affect the measurement of personality traits such as psychopathy. It appears that Hare's Psychopathy Checklist, whether in PCL-R or PCL-SV form, is valid for the comparison of women with each other but would not be valid for comparing men and women. One could be fairly confident that a woman with a score of 25 on the PCL-R would have higher levels of psychopathy than a woman with a score of 20, but it would not be appropriate to draw conclusions about the relative levels of psychopathy of a man with a score of 25 and a woman with a score of 20.

A further warning is necessary at this point, on the pitfalls of attempting to reduce any person to a single number. It would be wrong to assume that two people with the same score on the PCL-R are the same in any way other than their score, irrespective of whether they are men or women. There is more than one way to obtain the same numerical score, and ratings of this type are no substitute for a full assessment. Similar reservations apply to any psychological test, including the gold standard of intelligence testing; the fact that two people have the same IQ does not mean that they will be similar in any other way.

Although there are few differences in the principles of assessing risk in men and women, the management of risk is a different matter. There is a growing literature on the characteristics of forensic mental health services for women, but it falls beyond the scope of this text.

## Learning difficulties

Again, the principles of risk assessment are the same. Specialist skills come into play if communication difficulties complicate gathering of information, and the presence of learning difficulties can alter or mask the symptoms of other mental disorders.

The presence of learning difficulties may complicate specialized treatments because cognitive-behavioural programmes for violence reduction are usually designed for a population of normal intelligence. It is important to remember that this comment applies only to such specialist services, and most violence risk reduction in general mental health settings is achieved by the effective but straightforward management of mental disorder.

## Personality disorder

Personality disorder benefits from at least a degree of structure in relation to assessment and treatment. Without structure it can be difficult to pin down, as the nature of the problem, and the targets of treatment, are usually less clear than is the case with symptoms of mental illness. Depending on the context, one form or another of the Psychopathy Checklist is almost mandatory, and it would be a brave personality disorder service that did not use this instrument or an equivalent.

Drift is a major problem in personality disorder services, as staff lose sight of the main goals of treatment and find themselves side-tracked by other issues or crises. Standardized dynamic measures, such as the Violence Risk Scale (Wong and Gordon, 2000), are therefore useful in directing and monitoring treatment. As it requires training and time, its use tends to be confined to specialist services. The principle's of setting out clear goals at the start of treatment and keeping them in mind throughout, is good for all services.

Mental health workers, with some justification, often see personality disorder patients as being more difficult to assess and manage, but it can be argued that they are more predictable than the mentally ill. Even when there is impulsivity, the patient can be relied on to behave impulsively and unreliably. There is often a degree of continuity that is lost in some severely mentally ill patients, and psychotic behaviour is more likely to have a strong random element.

The continuities in personality disordered behaviour are important in risk management because, leaving aside fluctuations in crisis, risks generally persist over a long period of time. For this reason it is necessary to think very carefully before recommending the compulsory hospitalization of any patient with a pure personality disorder (i.e. a personality disorder without mental illness). And the thinking should be on the specific question of how they are going to leave hospital. If the risk is sufficient to require detention now, how and when will it change? Hospitalization is best kept as a short-term intervention for the management of risk at times of crisis. I would never recommend an open-ended hospital order for a mentally disordered offender with personality disorder alone.

Personality disorder, and psychopathy in particular, also raises questions of motivation and goals. Most medical treatment assumes common goals shared by patient and doctor, even if there is transient disturbance at times of severe mental illness. In psychopathy the patient may have deeply ingrained antisocial attitudes. He may not recognize the need for, or the desirability of, a strategy to reduce violence risk, and he may even take pride in his capacity for violence. There is an obvious dilemma for a service that is meant to have respect for the rights and views of users, while at the same time working to reduce risk. Solutions are difficult to find. Motivational interviewing may help to establish common ground but it cannot work miracles. Compulsory treatment is a massive step to take and should be contemplated only by specialist services.

## Summary: the application of structured clinical risk assessment

The structured clinical assessment of violence risk ensures that the decisions of a clinician are informed by, but not constrained by, specific background information. It is ultimately a clinical method. Its strength and its weakness it that it does not tell clinicians what to do but helps them to decide for themselves, and it aids communication about risk by encouraging use of a common language.

As it is a clinical method, it is best when used by an experienced team. When confronted by marginal decisions that are marginal, the solution will usually be the trusted clinical standby of the second opinion. The second opinion is an underused resource in violence risk management. It introduces the possibility of a fresh insight and, even if there is no revelation and the decision remains the same, it represents a sharing of the risk.

Chapter 7

# A new look at homicides by the mentally ill: applying structured risk assessment

Chapter 3 described the origins and development of the UK's homicide Inquiries. From the start they provoked a mixed response but, as the number of reports has proliferated, all parties have come to agree that the reports are becoming repetitive and there is a problem of diminishing returns. How many times can one repeat the call for better communication before recognizing the irony and searching for a better way to get the message across? The chapter ended with a summary of the new approach taken by the Confidential Inquiry into Suicides and Homicides (NCISH), and suggested that the individual reports will become less important in the future.

While independent Inquiries into homicides are becoming less important and may become less frequent, there is more to be learned from existing data. One problem is the gap between the detailed clinical information contained in independent Inquiry reports, and the rather bald statistics that emerge from NCISH. I have emphasized the stunning finding from NCISH that schizophrenia is found in 5% of homicide perpetrators compared with 1% of the general population (Shaw *et al.*, 2006), but the explanation of this association remains unclear. Was the mental illness coincidental? Did the killing come out of the blue, or was the risk apparent long before the event? Did problems in treatment contribute to the outcome? Were associated problems of substance misuse more important than the mental illness itself? Was the killing motivated by psychotic symptoms?

The answers to these questions will vary. Presumably some offences were related to treatment failures and some were not, so a statistical analysis may not be helpful. Independent Inquiry reports into each case would answer many of the questions but they are not the ideal solution. The NCISH and the independent Inquiries are at opposite ends of a spectrum. The NCISH is systematic and has comprehensive coverage of cases; the independent Inquiries are detailed but idiosyncratic, so it may be difficult to extract general lessons. The NCISH data are readily accessible and easy to interpret, whereas independent Inquiry reports are lengthy, time consuming to read, and more open to interpretation. For example, the lessons drawn by the chairman of an Inquiry may not be the lessons that would be drawn by a clinician, and they many not be clinically useful. Table 7.1 summarizes some of the advantages and disadvantages of the two approaches.

In scientific terms, Table 7.1 amounts to a summary of the differences between epidemiology and single case studies. The contest between those two methods is an unequal one, and from a scientific point of view it is tempting to dismiss the single case methodology entirely. But there is more than science involved. The values attached to these events mean that single cases are important. Service failures may not feature in most homicides so they are not prominent in the epidemiology, but as providers of services we need to know about them. The challenge is to find methods that include systematic analysis of data and detailed individual scrutiny of cases, without having to read and interpret a series of long, individual reports.

One solution proposed by the NCISH is to adapt the psychological autopsy technique that has been used by researchers to investigate the psychosocial aspects of suicide. Barraclough *et al.* (1974) is an early example of the use of this approach to extract clinical lessons from 100 suicides. Hawton *et al.* (1998) is a review of the methodological issues. The method is based on semistructured

**Table 7.1** Advantages and disadvantages of independent inquiry reports and the Confidential Inquiry into Suicides and Homicides (NCISH)

| Independent Inquiries | Confidential Inquiry |
| --- | --- |
| Individual, case-by-case approach | Uniform method applied to all cases |
| Idiosyncratic | Systematic |
| Mass of clinical detail | Brief summary of clinical information |
| Good on details of each case | Simplified account misses some details |
| Emphasis on individual motivations and performance | Details of motivation and performance may be missed |
| Details of one case | Accessible data from hundreds of cases |
| Time consuming to read | Can be read quickly |
| Broader associations may be missed | Specific problems missed |
| Findings may not be generalizable | Generalizable findings |

interviews with relevant individuals, after the event. It remains to be seen whether it will be possible to apply the same approach to homicides, and there are formidable obstacles in the current research climate. For example, ethical questions have been raised about whether it is acceptable for researchers even to write an initial letter to those who have committed a homicide.

Meanwhile, in another effort to extract all possible lessons from data collected by NCISH and from independent Inquiry reports, the Department of Health's Risk Management Programme Board commissioned a review of mental health homicides and Inquiry reports, which was carried out in early 2006. The review was an attempt to apply structured risk assessment techniques retrospectively. I will now describe the sample, method, and conclusions, ending with a summary of cases that illustrate particular points.

## Review of homicides by violent patients with severe mental illness

The intention was to review priority cases, consisting of those with a diagnosis of mental illness and a known history of violence. The review considered data from all available sources and had two guiding principles. The first was adherence to Root Cause Analysis, in that the main interest was in underlying, systemic or general factors rather than the actions of individuals. The second principle was the use of a structured clinical assessment of violence risk (SCAVR), using information available to the clinical team at the time of the homicide.

### The sample

The following criteria were used to extract a subset of cases from the database of the NCISH (see Chapter 3 for details):

1. A current patient of NHS mental health services in England and Wales committing a homicide during the last 10 years.
2. A diagnosis of 'Schizophrenia or other delusional disorder' or of 'Bipolar affective disorder' as recorded on the Homicide Form for the NCISH.
3. A history of previous violence known to the mental health team before the homicide occurred.
4. Availability of NCISH forms; at least one psychiatric court report; and, preferably, an independent Inquiry report relating to the homicide.

### Rationale for the case selection criteria

The aim was to concentrate on cases that should have been a priority for services, in that the patients had a major mental illness (almost always schizophrenia) and they had a known history of violence. The study concentrated on recent cases because policies and practice in this area have changed rapidly and older cases may not be relevant. On the other hand, the cases could not be too recent as it takes time for them to get into the system and for the criminal trial and Inquiry to be conducted.

## Description and analysis

Data were gathered from all available sources, including NCISH records, psychiatric reports prepared for the trial, independent Homicide Inquiry reports when available, and clinical records.

The data were used to complete the HCR20 (Historical Clinical Risk-20; Webster *et al.*, 1997) for each case. This structured clinical assessment of violence risk is described in detail in Chapter 6.

## The HCR20

The HCR20 has been widely used in clinical populations and is a standard assessment within many forensic psychiatry services in Canada and, to a growing extent, in the UK.

It consists of 10 Historical, five Clinical, and five Risk Management items relating to a patient. Each can be scored as definitely present, probably or partially present, or absent. A list of the items appears in Chapter 6.

In broad terms, the Historical, Clinical, and Risk Management groups relate to past, present, and future. The Historical items are concerned with past behaviour, personality, and mental illness. The Clinical items relate to current mental state and behaviour, and the Risk Management items relate to predicted functioning in the future.

## Demography of the sample

The NCISH provided data for all cases fitting the criteria from 1995 to 2002. On manual inspection and consideration of further reports, a few of the cases did not fit the criteria and were discarded. The reasons for removing cases were doubt over whether there was a known history of violence, and persisting doubt over the correct diagnostic category. Exclusion of such cases left 25, with offence dates ranging from November 1995 to December 2002.

### Ethnic origin

It emerged from a detailed review of the cases that at least two were marginal for inclusion in the sample because of doubts over whether the diagnosis or the history of violence were known to the service at the time. Both these cases

**Table 7.2** Ethnic origin of total sample (*n* = 25)

| Ethnic origin | No. | % |
|---|---|---|
| White | 16 | 68 |
| Black Caribbean | 4 | 16 |
| Black African | 2 | 8 |
| Indian/Pakistani/Bangladeshi | 1 | 4 |
| Other | 2 | 8 |
| Total | 25 | 100 |

are of white ethnic origin, so if they had been excluded by a strict application of the selection criteria the distribution of ethnic origin would be further skewed towards over-representation of minorities.

## HCR20 data: Historical items

This section of the HCR20 consists of 10 items in the history that are likely to be related to an increased risk of violence.

It should be noted that the sample selection criteria ensure that all cases have H1 (Previous Violence) and H6 (Major Mental Illness). The criteria are listed here to demonstrate that it is not unreasonable that a clinical team should have this sort of information available, particularly when there is a known history of violence.

**Table 7.3** Frequency distribution of HCR20 Historical items in the total sample (*n* = 25)

| No. of items present | No. | % |
|---|---|---|
| 10 | 10 | 40 |
| 9 | 4 | 16 |
| 8 | 1 | 4 |
| 7 | 6 | 24 |
| 6 | 2 | 8 |
| 5 | 2 | 8 |
| <5 | 0 | – |
| Total | 25 | 100 |

**Table 7.4** Frequency distribution of HCR20 Clinical items in the sample ($n = 25$)

| No. of items present | No. | % |
|---|---|---|
| 5 | 15 | 60 |
| 4 | 5 | 20 |
| 3 | 2 | 8 |
| 2 | 2 | 8 |
| 1 | 1 | 4 |
| 0 | – | – |
| Total | 25 | 100 |

## HCR20 data: Clinical items

The five Clinical items are listed in Chapter 6. As with the Historical items, it is reasonable to suppose that this sort of information should be available to the team. The frequency distribution for the Clinical items is shown in Table 7.4.

## HCR20 data: Risk Management items

The five Risk Management items are listed in Chapter 6. As they relate to future plans, it was more difficult to complete these items in retrospect, than was the case for the Historical and Clinical items. My point of reference for ratings was the last contact with the clinical team. Were there feasible plans, was there current or likely exposure to destabilizers or stress, was there any personal support, and was the patient compliant with whatever treatment was offered? These are, hopefully, the sorts of questions likely to be considered at a

**Table 7.5** Frequency distribution of HCR20 Risk Management items in the sample ($n = 25$)

| No. of items present | No. | % |
|---|---|---|
| 5 | 11 | 44 |
| 4 | 6 | 24 |
| 3 | 3 | 12 |
| 2 | 1 | 4 |
| 1 | 4 | 16 |
| 0 | – | – |
| Total | 25 | 100 |

care-planning meeting when dealing with a patient who has a history of violence. In most cases it was possible to make a rating.

## Preliminary discussion

### Overall numbers

The first point to make is that the number of cases is small, despite the fact that the study period spans 7 years. The average is less than four cases per annum. Of course there is more to this issue than simple numbers, but this figure must be seen in the context of other homicides. The overall homicide rate for England and Wales from 1995 to 1997 ranged from 584 to 650 cases per year, and by 2001/2002 it was close to 800 cases per annum. In other words, the cases with which we are concerned here account for less than half of 1% of all homicides in England and Wales. Even if the true number of cases was two or three times the number detected by NCISH, it is still a tiny proportion of all homicides. Frequency is not the same as importance, and one of this book's themes is that different values attach to different outcomes, so rare events may be very important. Even so, it is important to keep the problem in proportion.

### Ethnic origin

There is an over-representation of ethnic minorities relative to the general population. The marginal cases described above were both white British, so if they had been excluded the sample would have been more skewed.

The numbers are too small to draw any conclusions, but the data are obviously relevant to ongoing concern about possible over-representation of ethnic minorities among detained patients. At the very least, these figures are a reminder of the complexity of the issues involved (Singh and Burns, 2006).

### HCR20 data

The Historical items are important to the present study because they can be assessed reasonably accurately in retrospect. They concern aspects of the history that can be determined from the records. If the information can be obtained now, it could presumably have been obtained at the time. The information required to complete all these items was probably in the records before the homicide.

Ten of the 25 patients scored on all items of the H (Historical) scale, and 20 patients (80% of the sample) had seven or more items present. The HCR20 is not an actuarial scale, so adding up the scores is not necessarily a good indication of overall risk of violence. Even so, the presence in one patient of all or most of the Historical factors associated with increased violence risk is not to be dismissed lightly.

The importance of these cases is not that they must inevitably have a high, immediate risk of violence but that they are potentially a high risk. To use a gambling analogy, the stakes are high. That need not be a problem if the team is playing safe, but when there are also high Clinical and Risk Management scores the situation is worrying and ought to be given high priority. Even if one is cynical about the value of violence risk assessment, it is likely that any subsequent Inquiry into events will take into account these historical indicators of violence risk. The team ought to be aware of them so they walk into a high-risk situation with their eyes open, rather than learn about the risks after the event.

The findings for the Clinical and Risk scales were high for many of the patients. These figures may be less reliable when derived from records in retrospect, but this reservation should not be overstated. Items such as non-compliance, lack of response to treatment, or negative attitudes were usually easy to determine from records. In many cases complaints about these problems were all too frequent.

Also, errors arising from retrospective scoring will tend to understate the problem because the coding was based on the records. For example, lack of insight or the presence of symptoms may have been overlooked clinically whereas a systematic assessment would have revealed them. In other words, these are minimum estimates and could well have been higher if the systematic assessment had been done at the time.

As with the Historical ratings, the Clinical and Risk Management scores tend to be at the high end of the scale. Even though high ratings do not equate to high risk, many of these cases are impressive in having all or most of the factors that tend to predict violence risk. On this basis, homicides by the severely mentally ill are far from random events that could happen in any patient. Looked at in terms of violence risk indicators, many of these cases were extraordinary patients before the homicide.

The flaw in this reasoning is that such scores may be common in patients looked after in the community. Use of the HCR20 has been limited in the UK, but early results from research at the Institute of Psychiatry based on patients in south London suggests that forensic community patients generally score high on the H items of the HCR20, whereas many patients in general services score highly on C or R items, but high scores on all three are unusual (Fahy, personal communication). Most of the patients in the present sample resemble forensic patients in terms of their HCR ratings, although few were under the care of a forensic service.

## Would structured clinical risk assessment have made a difference to the outcome?

A definitive answer to the crucial question is impossible from a study of this type. Still, a reasonable estimate can be given, based on the following assumptions.

The first assumption is that the clinical team was not giving the case the priority it deserved. In some cases there was an awareness of the high risks involved but the team felt they could not do more under present legislation. More information about risk would not have made a difference here, as it would have re-stated what the team already knew. On the other hand there were plenty of cases in which the team did not recognize high risks.

The second assumption, in cases where the risk was not recognized, is that the team would have been more cautious in management of the case if it had seen a stark assessment of the violence risks involved. Considering the emphasis on risk since 1994, it would be comforting to find an automatic link between risk assessment and attempts at risk management. The reality is more worrying, as some of the following case vignettes show.

## Case summaries from review of homicides

### Note on the case summaries

After much thought, I have left out names and locations. All this information is in the public domain but repetition of the names involved may further stigmatize the patients concerned and hamper rehabilitation, as well as causing further distress to relations and professionals. As it was necessary to include circumstantial detail to illustrate particular points it is inevitable that some of the cases can be identified by those who are familiar with the circumstances, whether from personal involvement or by reading press or Inquiry reports.

The case numbers are arbitrary and the given age was that at the time of the offence unless otherwise specified. I have attempted to summarize the main issues at the beginning of each case, but this is not meant to be an exhaustive account of all the lessons that can be drawn from a case.

---

### Case 2

HCR20 Scores: H = 10, C = 5, R = 5.

**Main issues:** Killing of a stranger for psychotic motives; family history of violent and antisocial behaviour; violence and personality disorder before onset of illness; extensive and serious criminality unrelated to illness; non-compliance; drug and alcohol misuse; team recognized extent of violence risk and made efforts to control it within existing powers; forensic services were involved; little more could have been done; role for community treatment order.

---

This 29-year-old man was from a family with a long and extensive history of violent and antisocial behaviour. He had been in contact with services for several years, during which time he had been given diagnoses of schizophrenia, personality disorder, and drug and alcohol abuse. There was a long history of offending including serious violence (stabbings) both when psychotic and when well. There were several admissions with rapid remission of psychotic symptoms on medication, then a refusal to take depot after discharge, followed by relapse in the community. There was close monitoring of the case, including use of a supervision order, and there was a detailed assessment of his mental state only a few days before the offence. Although a general psychiatry team looked him after, they had sought and followed the advice of the forensic psychiatry team.

The offence was the apparently motiveless killing of a stranger. The clinicians concerned, and the Inquiry, concluded that little more could be done without the power to enforce medication while the patient was in the community.

**Comment** Structured clinical risk assessment would not have made a difference. The risks were recognized and managed as well as possible under existing law. This case is as close as one gets to seeing clinicians struggling against the limits of what is possible in risk management. Note, however, that the problem clinicians struggled with was not the assessment of the violence risk, on which all were agreed, but the limited powers available to manage that risk. Although the outcome was negative, there was no criticism of the clinical team in the Inquiry report.

---

## Case 27

HCR20 Scores: H = 10, C = 5, R = 5

**Main issues:** Killing of his mother while floridly psychotic; violence and personality disorder before onset of illness; extensive and serious criminality unrelated to illness; poor continuing care after initial treatment of psychosis in prison; non-compliance; drug misuse; missed opportunity to recommend restriction order after previous violent offence; failure to appreciate extent of violence risk; managed by general services in community despite previous forensic involvement; possible role for community treatment order.

---

The patient's personal history is uncertain but he was brought up partly in the UK and partly in Nigeria. From the age of 12 he was in the UK. He truanted, got into a lot of fights at school and was expelled. He smoked cannabis from the age of 15 years and would come and go as he pleased at home, despite his parents' best efforts to control him.

He had no qualifications and was soon involved in criminal activity. While attending college he stabbed a fellow student, supposedly in a fight over drug dealing, and left within 2 months of starting his course. He was later given a 4-year sentence for the offence of wounding.

He was unemployed for some years and never held a job for any length of time. He was promiscuous and may have had children he did not see or support. He had no steady relationships.

In February 1996 he was given a 4½-year sentence for robbery. He approached a car, forced the driver out, punched him, and stole his keys. He was not mentally ill. His motivation was the desire for money to buy cocaine. During his sentence he suffered a psychotic breakdown and was transferred to a medium secure forensic unit in January 1997. He responded to medication and returned to prison in August 1997. He had to be transferred in April 1999 after a further breakdown, this time to a forensic unit in the independent sector because no beds were available in his local unit. He was transferred only 4 days before the end of his sentence so he had the status of an ordinary, detained patient almost immediately after his arrival at the hospital. This meant he was not subject to a restriction order so it was not possible to place conditions on his eventual release to the community.

He committed a serious assault within the forensic unit in September 1999, when he threw hot water in the face of another patient who had alleged to staff that he was using cannabis. He was transferred to his local locked ward later in September but was still unwell. Soon after arrival he fondled a female nurse and continued to use cannabis.

In November 1999 he was convicted of causing actual bodily harm for the offence committed in the forensic unit. He was sentenced to detention under a Hospital Order, which was rather pointless as he was already detained under such an order. He was transferred to an open ward in January 2000 then promptly went absent without leave, along with another patient.

He was discharged to his mother's home in June 2000 and placed on the Supervision Register. He was doing well on depot medication but discontinued it in August 2000 in favour of oral olanzapine.

His last contact with services was on 14 March 2001 when he was seen in the outpatient department. He was relaxed and friendly but non-compliant with his oral medication. He described frequent arguments with his mother. He was not seen again until after he killed his mother in May 2001.

On the day of the killing his brother called the police. The patient had stabbed his mother and appeared psychotic. His reported statements included: 'I'm going to be king of the world … she's evil …' There was a previous history of threats to his mother and his brother.

**Comment** This man had a well-established history as a violent criminal before he developed a mental illness. He had a severe personality disorder before he became mentally ill. After the onset of mental illness he was never compelled to comply with medication in the community. Forensic services were involved but never took long-term responsibility for the case and the patient returned to the community through general services.

There was a strong case in favour of forensic services managing his care because his mental illness first became apparent during a long prison sentence for violence, and there were obvious risks. Structured assessment would have made those risks explicit. A community treatment order would have been useful but there was also a missed opportunity to recommend a restriction order following the assault in the medium secure unit. The case raises many issues, including follow-up of patients transferred back to prison after treatment in medium security, because there was no real continuity of care.

## Case 19

HCR20 Scores: H = 10, C = 5, R = 5

**Main issues:** Killing of fellow patient on ward with no apparent motive; violence and personality disorder before onset of illness; failure to appreciate extent of violence risk, even with hindsight; enforcement of ward policies; alcohol use on ward; need for structured clinical assessment of violence risk.

This 26-year-old man had a history of poor parenting and a miserable childhood. There was physical and emotional abuse, much of it related to his father's alcoholism, although his mother was also violent. His first conviction was for assault occasioning actual bodily harm aged 13 years, when he shot someone with an air rifle. There were frequent changes of school. He never settled, and he truanted frequently. He was expelled from school for robbery aged 15 years and soon became a heavy user of amphetamines and cannabis.

He had paramilitary interests and often wore Nazi clothing or memorabilia. He was known to collect knives and, unknown to staff, had a set of chef's knives with him in the hospital on the admission during which he killed a fellow patient. He had never worked as a chef.

He was diagnosed as suffering from paranoid schizophrenia at the age of 20 years. Over the 5-year period of contact with mental health services he had many admissions, usually associated with amphetamine abuse. He was placed on the supervision register because of concerns about the safety of his mother, whom he had repeatedly intimidated. He was said to be a loner but he was usually polite and not threatening with staff and fellow patients.

In December 1998 he attacked and killed a fellow patient in the hospital where he had been admitted earlier that month. The attack was unprovoked and unpredictable. The patient was lying on his bed and the victim was simply the next person to enter the room. There was no context of animosity or conflict between the two men. The perpetrator had a row with another patient earlier in the day and seems to have confused the two men in a muddled way reflective of psychotic thinking. The patient was never able to give a satisfactory account of his motivation. He had been drinking earlier that day. Also, he had been wearing his German military uniform on the ward, which had upset some of the other patients and appears to have contributed to his sense of paranoia, in that there were genuine feelings of anger and hostility towards him.

His consultant described the admission to hospital as 'a social admission': he had been made homeless from his hostel after allegedly committing a burglary. He was compliant with medication during the admission 'for the first time in months'. The consultant also commented that there was 'no track record of violence'. Even after the offence, the consultant's evidence to the Inquiry was that the patient presented a low risk of violence.

The patient said he had taken no illicit drugs for a week (at other times he said a month) before the offence. On remand he was transferred to a high security hospital and settled, later showing no psychotic symptoms when free of medication. Reports agreed he suffered from a severe personality disorder but were equivocal on the question of mental illness and its role in the offence.

**Comment** There are two main issues for prevention, both of which were emphasized in the Inquiry report. First, there is the question of nursing practice and maintaining a safe ward environment. The patient habitually dressed in a German uniform with Nazi regalia and, although he was generally polite, this is hardly acceptable conduct on a ward where it is bound to cause offence. He drank heavily on the ward on several occasions, and he was able to bring in a set of chef's knives. The message is that basic ward procedures go a long way to ensuring a safe and secure environment, even though one could not predict that breach of those procedures would lead to a serious violent incident.

The second major issue concerns diagnosis and the management of violence risk. The patient had a working diagnosis of schizophrenia so the post-offence re-assessment is largely irrelevant. The violence risk assessment in this case seems not to have gone beyond the fact that he had never done anything like this before and his mental state was much the same as usual. Such information is relevant but not sufficient for a proper risk assessment. A structured clinical assessment of risk would have shown that this patient ticked all the boxes for violence risk. The offence could not have been predicted but the patient's potential for violence would have been better appreciated. There were sufficient indications to justify the fuller assessment of violence risk, including the fact he had been placed on the Supervision Register because of the risk of violence to his mother.

The most telling aspect of this case is the consultant's insistence, even after the killing, that there were no indications of violence risk. This is simply not true, as the HCR20 ratings and the history of threatened and actual violence show. It is bizarre to argue that an admission is 'for social reasons' when it was precipitated by the patient's offending leading to him being evicted. This incident raises two concerns; first that the offending is evidence of a deterioration in mental state; and second that the loss of accommodation leads to instability, uncertainty, and a loss of social supports. None of this meant he was about to kill someone, but it was all bad news in terms of violence risk.

One is forced to conclude that, when discussing violence risk, the professionals working in this service literally 'did not know what they were talking about'. They did not have the concepts or language needed to give a proper description of the violence risks. That conclusion is not meant as a criticism of the individuals involved, but they were out of their depth in managing a patient with so many indicators of violence risk. This is unacceptable for all concerned, and not least for the team who were left vulnerable to criticism in relation to an offence that could not have been predicted.

## Case 17

HCR20 Scores: H = 7, C = 5, R = 5

**Main issues:** Killing of a stranger arising directly from psychotic symptoms; normal before onset of illness; extensive violence and drug use after onset of illness; homelessness; non-compliance; delay in intervention despite obvious deterioration; possible benefits of community treatment order.

The patient was born in the UK to Jamaican parents. He had an unremarkable childhood and completed secondary education, his only problem being truancy in his last 2 years. He left at 16 with a few CSE exam passes and went on to have a good work record in skilled manual jobs until he became mentally ill at the age of 19 years.

There were a couple of minor offences in his late teens but his offending escalated after the onset of his mental illness. Aged 26 he was arrested for stabbing a female acquaintance and set fire to his cell when on remand, resulting in his transfer to a medium secure forensic unit. He was discharged to a hostel a few weeks later in January 1995, having been sentenced to probation with a condition of psychiatric treatment. The Inquiry was later to criticize this disposal, on the grounds that a Hospital Order with restrictions would have been more appropriate to such a serious offence.

While on probation he was generally compliant with depot medication but also generally uncommunicative. When the probation order ended in August 1995 he went to live with his mother. In September 1997 he stopped all medication, having been grudgingly and partially compliant until then. He was often withdrawn, socially isolated, and apathetic. A Community Psychiatric Nurse (CPN) continued to visit him after he stopped taking his medication.

By early December 1997 he was relapsing with signs of hypomania and, after voluntary admission ended with his impulsive decision to discharge himself, he was detained on 15 December as a civil patient under Section 3 of the Mental Health Act 1983. His mother disagreed with the compulsory admission and had to be displaced as nearest relative.

During the later part of this admission, while at home on leave, he set fire to his car and burned himself, in an inept attempt to defraud the insurance company. This incident was thought to reflect his impaired judgement. In April 1998 he became violent when told he would have to take depot medication and it was necessary to call in the police to restrain him after he produced a screwdriver and threatened staff. He was transferred to a medium secure unit and showed no insight into his illness or the seriousness of this incident.

He was discharged from the medium secure unit in December 1998 with a diagnosis of bipolar affective disorder and paranoid personality disorder. His medication was carbamazepine (a mood stabilizer) and risperidone (an antipsychotic) both given orally. There had been real difficulties with his depot medication. Earlier objections had been based on weight gain, and he later developed breasts as a side-effect, to such an extent that surgical intervention was considered.

There were difficulties with his outpatient attendance soon after discharge and by February 1999 he was saying he wanted to sever all links with mental health services. Staff persuaded him to stay in touch but in July 1999 he reported he had not taken any oral medication for about 6 months. He was again asking to break off all contact with services. His supervising consultant, a forensic psychiatrist, could find no definite signs of relapse. After discussion among the team there was contact with the patient's GP because of concerns that he may relapse in the immediate future. The seriousness of the situation was recognized by the psychiatrist, who consulted his medical defence society about his personal position.

On 6 August 1999 the patient telephoned his consultant and asked to have access to his medical records. Although there were no other apparent signs of relapse apparent during the call, such a demand was known to be a possible early indicator of relapse in this patient. It emerged after the event that there had been several odd interactions with the GP around this time e.g. when the patient asked the GP to remove from his records all references to mental illness. The patient had also been to the police station to complain that hospital staff were following him around, but this information was not passed on to the team. The Inquiry details several failures of communication and of procedure relating to the Care Programme Approach.

The homicide took place on 11 August 1999. The night before, the patient's sister had noted his wild demeanour. He presented at a general hospital during the early hours, complaining of sleeplessness and overactivity but not waiting to be assessed. Later that day he attacked and killed a stranger, an elderly man, immediately after he had stabbed a 12-year-old child and his father. The latter two victims survived but these offences were attempted murders. There was no interaction between victims and perpetrator before the homicidal attacks. He attacked the police who arrested him and was found to have started a fire and left the gas on at his flat, where he was restrained and arrested. The patient later linked his offences to an impending solar eclipse. He believed the world was going to end and others were going to attack him so he had to get them first.

**Comment** This is an example of the archetypal 'killing of a stranger' (see below under Discussion). In general terms, it is also a case in which there was a known violence risk that was not managed effectively. There were plenty of opportunities for earlier intervention and one of the lessons of the case is, in simple terms, that there is no need to wait for a florid relapse when a patient with a history of violence is non-compliant and allowing restricted access to his mental state. The previous stabbing was an indicator of what was potentially at stake here, and there was too great a reluctance to intervene. If the case is worrying enough to prompt a call to the consultant's defence union, it must at least warrant a Mental Health Act assessment.

Although a high risk was recognized, a structured clinical assessment may have been helpful. It would have made explicit the fact that, in a person with a history of serious violence, all the Clinical and Risk Management indicators were positive (reflected in the scores above of C = 5 and R = 5). The service proceeded on the basis that there were no grounds for detention but an explicit statement of the risk factors would have begged the question: if detention is not justified in a patient who ticks all the risk boxes, when is it justified?

The Inquiry pointed up many failures in communication and procedure but it is useful to look behind these operational or tactical issues to consider the overall strategy for managing violence risk in this case. The strategy was to monitor closely the mental state and intervene early in a florid relapse. Yet this was a patient who had never been forthcoming about his inner thoughts even when he was forced to comply. He was now refusing medication, had a recent history of covert non-compliance, and wanted no further contact with mental health services. He was willing to see his GP but only on the understanding that he had physical problems and his mental health was good—so much so that he demanded any reference to previous problems should be removed from the records. In other words, there had never been full access to his thoughts and it became virtually non-existent, so the only guide to his mental state was his behaviour—which was rarely observed.

In these circumstances, operational and procedural concerns miss the point. Monitoring was not an adequate strategy because of the limited access to his mental state, and it could never have contained the violence risk. As the mental state changes rapidly, and symptoms may be hidden at an interview, a reassuring presentation one day does not exclude the possibility of serious violence the next day, or even hours later. Close monitoring is not an adequate strategy for containing such a risk in the community and mental health staff are left in a difficult position when they rely on it (hence the consultant's call to the defence union before the homicide).

The correct and inescapable strategy for managing the violence risk in this case was enforced compliance with medication. How could this have been achieved?

The Inquiry was critical of the failure to impose a Hospital Order with restrictions after an earlier stabbing. This comment has been made before by several homicide Inquiries, so much so that it has become a well-worn subject of debate. The issues here were the usual ones. The Crown Prosecution Service (CPS) reduced the original charges to less serious ones because the patient was so obviously mentally ill (he was unfit to appear in court on two occasions). The patient's mental state improved with treatment, so by the time the case came to court there was no indication for inpatient treatment and the law did not allow compulsory treatment in the community.

Better liaison between agencies may help, and there are ongoing discussions on the related topic of prosecuting patients for offences committed while they are in hospital. The advent of Multi-Agency Public Protection Panels (MAPPPs) also promises better co-ordination. However, none of these developments addresses the fundamental problem. This patient needed treatment for his mental illness but he did not need to be detained in hospital once he was taking medication. There is also an argument against the criminalization of the mentally ill when offending is so clearly linked with psychotic symptoms, with no understandable motivation. The criminal justice system is based on notions of free will and moral choice and there will always be misgivings about labelling as a criminal a man whose violence derives from a malfunction of the brain.

This reluctance to criminalize the mentally ill is one of the positive aspects of our medico-legal system compared with that in the USA, and we should not abandon it completely. At the risk of repetition, the solution to this issue is surely a Community Treatment Order. Had one been in existence, the team concerned would almost certainly have used it to enforce compliance with medication and these attacks would not have happened.

---

## Case 8

HCR20 Scores: H = 6, C = 5, R = 5

**Main issues:** Killing of a stranger arising directly from psychotic symptoms; normal before onset of illness; extensive violence and drug use after onset of illness; homelessness; extensive past efforts to manage violence risk, but possible failure to appreciate extent of violence risk; non-compliance; delay in intervention despite obvious deterioration; possible benefits of community treatment order.

---

This 30-year-old man was essentially a normal student with an unremarkable family and childhood until he developed schizophrenia when he was 20 years old. The mental illness was of insidious onset and became severe. He was never well again after the first episode. He was never able to work, he had limited insight and he rarely complied with medication.

Although not violent before he developed schizophrenia, he was often violent when unwell. He had a well-documented history of attacks on fellow patients and on strangers. He had been on a Guardianship Order in an attempt to exert more control over his treatment in the community. He was a regular user of cannabis and another herbal drug.

The offence occurred in October 1997 after he had stopped his depot medication in March of that year because it interfered with his sexuality. He was given oral medication but did not take it. His mental state was deteriorating for months before the killing, with many reports of bizarre, threatening and aggressive behaviour. He lost accommodation several times because of his odd behaviour, once because he set a fire in a hotel room. He was homeless in the months leading up to the offence. Social workers tried to find accommodation but he invariably lost it because of his behaviour.

The offence occurred when the police attempted to arrest him in his flat, in a planned response to his deteriorating mental state and threatening behaviour. He stabbed and killed one of the officers as they broke into his flat, acting on the delusional belief that they planned to rape him.

The Inquiry recommended tighter supervision and better attempts to increase compliance. The media focused on the Inquiry's mention of incidents such as a GP once sending him medication in the post.

**Comment** The Inquiry stopped short of recommending compulsory treatment in the community but it is hard to see why. The patient's history of previous violence included unprovoked attacks on strangers and elderly, vulnerable people, and these offences would probably have been enough to warrant a restriction order in other circumstances.

The HCR20 assessment is complicated because of the early onset of mental illness. He does not score on historical variables relating to childhood disturbance, early violence and personality disorder/psychopathy. A case could be made for the latter two, as he functioned throughout his adult life as a man with a personality disorder, but conventional practice is not to use personality disorder as a label when the personality change is clearly related to serious mental illness.

This is a case that illustrates why the HCR20 is not just about adding up numbers. He achieves the maximum rating on Clinical and Risk variables, which in conjunction with his history of serious violence identifies him as a high risk of serious violence when mentally ill. An assessment of this type would have made the risks explicit and would have encouraged the tighter supervision recommended by the Inquiry.

It is hard to avoid the additional conclusion that the key to safe management of this case was compulsory treatment in the community. When his history of violence, drug misuse and lack of insight is taken into account, the Inquiry's recommendations for encouraging compliance appear unrealistic in their optimism.

Conflicting principles bear on this case. Here was a patient from an ethnic minority refusing medication for a clearly stated, potentially valid reason: it interfered with his sexual potency. Knowing he went on to kill, it is easy to say that mental health services should have overridden his wishes, but without the help of hindsight the decision is more difficult. Either we want mental health services to respect patient autonomy or we do not. If the former, then they should not lightly go against a patient's wishes and it seems right that it should be a matter for a Tribunal when they want to impose medication on a man who does not want to take it.

This may be a minority opinion and it is not my role to repeat the Inquiry, and certainly not to claim that I can do a better job. Perhaps the way forward is for there to be a wider debate about when a patient's past violence reaches a point at which compliance becomes a matter of the public interest, rather than simply a matter for the patient and the doctor?

MAPPPs may be relevant here and it seems likely that a patient of this type would now be referred to the local MAPPP. Even with MAPPP involvement, it is hard to see how this patient could be properly managed without the power to compel compliance with medication. The debate about when services should take control is rather academic if they lack the power to do so.

Case 8 is another example of a killing of a stranger. As with Case 17, there was no real history of personality disorder or violence before the onset of the mental illness. These cases serve as a reminder that schizophrenia alone can lead to a high risk of serious violence, with no relevant pre-morbid history. They are discussed at greater length below, when considering the evidence for and against two types of violence in schizophrenia.

---

### Case 25

HCR20 Scores: H = 7, C = 4, R = 4

**Main issues:** Homicide by a treated patient on a restriction order; homicide arising directly from psychotic symptoms; little antisocial behaviour before onset of illness; extensive violent offending and drug use after onset of illness; co-morbid cannabis use known to be associated with deterioration in mental state; failure of services to appreciate extent of violence risk; failure to intervene despite known positive symptoms and continuing use of cannabis over a long period.

---

This 40-year-old man had an uneventful childhood and first became mentally ill at the age of 21 years in 1982. In 1986 he attacked and threatened to kill a female police officer when he was mentally unwell.

He was placed on a Hospital Order with restrictions in 1993 for offences of arson and possession of a controlled drug with intent to supply. He set at least seven fires over a 3-year period, some of which were related to deterioration in his mental state brought about by smoking cannabis. He spent several years in a medium secure unit before being conditionally discharged in July 1997. He was often violent during the admission.

The offence took place in 2002 at the hostel where he had lived for 5 years. He attacked an elderly fellow resident for no apparent reason, grabbing him from behind without warning and cutting his throat. There was no history of bad feeling between them.

The patient was well known to staff and to those supervising him in the community. He was known within the hostel as a man who was sometimes sullen and often talked or laughed to himself. The main issue in his supervision had been his continuing use of cannabis. The team were concerned about it and had instituted urine checks 'as a baseline' but they were always positive. There had been a brief re-admission due to cannabis use in 1997 and he had been asked to leave the hostel in 1998 because of continuing cannabis use.

In July 2000 the team recommended a move to his own flat, despite continuing use of cannabis. This attempt at independent living failed about a year before the offence when his mental state deteriorated, probably because he was using a lot of cannabis. The failed attempt at independent living ended in a brief re-admission to hospital as a voluntary patient, and he then returned to the hostel at which he was well known.

He was compliant with prescribed medication but, as noted above, there were persistent abnormalities in his mental state. An account from the hostel manager described him as often being awake all night, sitting talking to himself, staring into space, and showing poor concentration. Another resident had complained he was banging on doors on the night before the offence.

The patient reported later that he had been thinking of killing somebody for 2 weeks, so he went to a shop and bought a knife. There was no explanation of his motivation or his choice of victim.

**Comment** This is an extraordinary case, particularly as it concerned a restricted patient. The main concern throughout several years in the community was continuing use of cannabis, which was involved in the offences that led to the restriction order in the first place and contributed to the failure of an attempt at independent living. Given that his mental state was never normal and his urine tests were never free of cannabis, it is difficult to understand why the team, or the Mental Health Unit of the Home Office, tolerated this situation. The most likely explanation appears to be that the personnel involved had become used to this odd scenario over a long period of time.

While the attack on a fellow resident was not predictable, the continuing disturbed mental state and use of cannabis together amounted to an unacceptable risk in view of the history. Part of the problem seems to have been that the team just got used to the patient and to his drug use.

Structured assessment of violence risk may have helped by leading to an explicit statement of the risk factors in this case. Those risk factors now look stark, and all the necessary information was available beforehand. One of the benefits of a formal, structured assessment of violence risk is that it amounts to a stocktaking exercise in patients who have been known to the team for a long time, and may drift into situations that appear worrying when looked at afresh.

Even so, the main issues in this case concern ethics, monitoring and intervention. Is it acceptable for a conditionally discharged restricted patient to continue to misuse cannabis when his mental state is abnormal and cannabis is known to make it worse? My answer would be no, and there should be a wider ethical debate about such issues.

The monitoring in this case was good, but the lack of intervention appears extraordinary with the benefit of hindsight. The team were spectators to deterioration when they should have been in control of the situation.

## Case 6

HCR20 Scores: H = 10, C = 5, R = 5

**Main issues:** Offending before onset of illness; co-morbid drug use and personality disorder; preoccupation with diagnosis and failure of services to appreciate extent of violence risk; non-compliance and loss of contact with services; possible benefits of community treatment order.

This 31-year-old man showed behavioural problems from an early age, having grown up in an atmosphere of marital discord and excessive physical punishment amounting to physical abuse. By the age of 13 he showed mood swings and serious violent behaviour, leading to a conviction for breaking the jaw of another boy at school. Shortly afterwards he caused a scalp wound to a girl at school and was placed on a care order. Further violence led to placement at boarding school, where there was some improvement.

He had an unstable and unsettled existence after leaving school, moving between his parents' house, youth custody, hospital, bed and breakfast, hostels, and sleeping rough. He had many short-term relationships, often marked by conflict and violence.

He used cannabis regularly over many years and alcohol intermittently. Cannabis was blamed for several deteriorations in his mental state. From 1984 he had psychotic symptoms on occasion. By 1987 at least one psychiatrist had diagnosed schizophrenia, noting that his symptoms were 'made worse by cannabis and made better by antipsychotic medication'. Another psychiatrist concluded he was unsuitable for treatment because he suffered from a personality disorder.

In 1993 the GP requested an urgent assessment when the patient's girlfriend said he was getting violent and was likely to kill someone. The locum consultant who saw him at home noted 'a mild degree of psychosis' that may be drug-induced. He was detained in hospital on Section 2 shortly afterwards. There followed 4 years of intermittent contact with services, often after his arrest for offences including threatening behaviour, minor assaults, and indecent exposure. He was rarely free of symptoms, and he was usually uncooperative and non-compliant with his oral medication. He continued to smoke cannabis regularly. He was sometimes considered not to be detainable, for unspecified reasons, even though psychotic.

In December 1996 his GP struck him off his list. In early January 1997 social services closed the case after noting he had declined help since August of 1996. The homicide occurred later in January 1997. The victim was a pregnant woman with whom he was having a relationship. She died of head injuries but he denied involvement, despite overwhelming evidence, so the circumstances and motive remain unclear.

On remand he was floridly psychotic and he was transferred to a high security hospital.

**Comment** Structured clinical assessment of violence risk could have helped because the care given to this man was unsatisfactory in many ways. There was no attempt to manage the case proactively, nor was there any attempt to address the risks posed.

A major problem was the diagnosis of drug-induced psychosis, which acted as an excuse for inaction by mental health services. This issue will be discussed in more detail in a later section of this report. Personality disorder was also used as a reason for not providing treatment. The fact remains that the diagnosis of schizophrenia was made 10 years before the homicide, and the patient spent much of the intervening period in a psychotic state that was recognized by most psychiatrists who saw him.

A structured clinical assessment of risk would have drawn attention to the fact that this was a man who ticked all the boxes for violence risk. This is arguably more relevant and useful information than any particular diagnostic label.

In the background is the issue of compulsory treatment in the community, and he was never a good candidate for voluntary treatment. However, the limit of what could be achieved through persuasion was never reached in this case because of the laissez-faire approach to his treatment.

## Case 3
HCR20 Scores: H = 10, C = 3, R = 2

**Main issues:** Drunken killing of an acquaintance; violence and personality disorder before onset of illness; alcohol misuse; reasonable level of care and mental state stable at time of offence; no direct link between illness and offence; alcohol as a cause of violence.

This 30-year-old man had over 10 years of contact with services with three well established diagnoses: schizo-affective disorder; severe personality disorder; and drug and alcohol misuse. He led an unstable life with frequent offending but his mental illness was under control at the time of the offence. He had a 2-day admission just days before the offence but was judged free of symptoms of mental illness.

The offence was a fight with an acquaintance late at night when both had been drinking. The patient had consumed more than 10 pints of beer that night but had a good memory for events. According to witnesses and his account, no symptoms of mental illness were apparent at the time. He did not appear unwell when arrested and he remained free of symptoms when assessed on remand. Court reports agreed there was no direct link between his mental illness and the offence. They agreed that his antisocial personality and his excessive drinking were relevant to the offence.

**Comment** Structured clinical risk assessment would not have made a difference. He was receiving a reasonable level of care in line with his current mental state and the killing bore no direct relationship to his mental illness. This is another example of the type of violence that featured heavily in the MacArthur study, in that the patient was behaving like others in his social circle by getting drunk and fighting.

---

### Case 24
HCR20 Scores: H = 9, C = 2, R = 1

**Main issues:** Offending before onset of illness; co-morbid drug addiction; homicide despite compliance with treatment and stable mental state; social influences on homicide; alcohol as a factor in violence.

---

This 29-year-old man had behavioural problems in childhood, including fighting, which led to his expulsion from school. He went on to acquire several criminal convictions before the emergence of his mental illness. His offending was mainly drug-related. He was discharged from the army in 1993 for smoking cannabis, and he was later imprisoned for importing cannabis and cocaine. He became addicted to heroin and was treated with methadone but found it difficult to comply with the regimen and used additional drugs. He developed hepatitis, which caused him a lot of anxiety.

He presented with psychotic symptoms in April 1997, having cut his arm 'to get the demons out'. During that first admission he assaulted another patient and a member of staff, following which he was taken away by the police and discharged as showing no signs of mental illness. In November 1997 he was seen in outpatients and noted to have been hearing voices for 2 years. He was prescribed oral antipsychotic medication. In July 1998 another consultant reinterpreted his symptoms as due to personality disorder and cannabis use, but continued to prescribe oral antipsychotic medication and a mood stabilizer. This is the acceptable face of re-diagnosis, in which the consultant makes a new diagnosis but continues to treat the old one just in case.

The patient was discharged from the clinic but a CPN saw him intermittently. He was still taking both medications when seen in November 1999, having drifted out of contact when he changed address. In March 2000 he was noted to have stopped his antipsychotic medication and his symptoms had returned. The medication was restarted and over the next 2 years the picture was dominated by his dependence on heroin, his struggles with the methadone regimen, and the diagnosis of hepatitis B in March 2001. He was often anxious but never floridly psychotic. His compliance with oral medication was good and he was motivated to comply by his expressed fear of becoming psychotic.

The offence occurred shortly after Christmas on 27 December. He had been drinking heavily in the pub with friends when he was encouraged by others to join an attack on a man said to be a paedophile. He went to the man's house with others, then beat him up and stabbed him. His family said his mental state had been stable in the weeks leading up to the killing. There was no evidence of delusions or hallucinations at the time of the killing. He was last seen by services a couple of weeks before the offence and there were no concerns. He became floridly psychotic while in prison on remand.

**Comment** In this case the mental illness appears to have been peripheral to the homicide. Also, his main problem in the years before the homicide was opiate addiction rather than schizophrenia, as his mental illness was well controlled by oral medication with which he was compliant. It is not clear that a structured assessment of violence risk would have made any difference to management of this case. The psychiatric care was of a reasonable standard and appears to have had no direct bearing on the outcome.

Although the offence was more serious than anything in that study, this is a good illustration of the type of violence that made up most of the incidents in the MacArthur study. Psychotic symptoms were not directly involved and the attack was related to the consumption of alcohol, along with social influences.

Perhaps most importantly, it seems unlikely that treatment could have prevented this incident. This theme is explored in more detail below, when considering different types of violence.

## Discussion and recommendations arising from the review of homicides

Structured clinical assessment of violence risk is a useful framework for looking at homicides by psychiatric patients. The value of the HCR20 in this study was that it got around some of the problems relating to hindsight, by introducing objectivity to the process. The Historical items are of most value in this respect. Characteristics such as 'Previous Violence' (H1), 'Young Age at First Violent Incident' (H2), 'Relationship Problems' (H3), 'Employment Problems' (H4), or 'Substance Use Problems' (H5) are not altered by hindsight.

The only way in which hindsight is likely to elevate ratings is if the homicide leads to the collection of data that was not available before. It is one of the cruel ironies of a homicide Inquiry that hundreds of thousands of pounds are expended on the collection of detailed information about a patient, when the service looking after him did not have the resources to gather data from so many sources. By contrast, the HCR20 relies on a limited set of variables and the data required ought to be available to any team looking after a patient with a history of violence. For example, the Clinical Items are: Lack of Insight; Negative Attitudes; Active Symptoms of Major Mental Illness; Impulsivity; and Unresponsiveness to Treatment. If the team are unable to assess these features of a case, they are in no position to address risk.

The following sections are presented under headings reflecting themes that emerged from the cases in the study.

## Schizophrenia as a cause of violence

The following discussion will emphasize the spectrum of influences on violence risk but we should not overlook the obvious. In at least 15 of these 25 cases, the motivation for the homicide was to be found mainly or solely in psychotic symptoms such as delusions or hallucinations. I have not included in this number those patients in whom disinhibition, impulsivity, or emotional lability arising from psychosis may have been important.

This finding does not and should not make comfortable reading for services. On the face of it, and despite the known history of violence, better control of the positive symptoms of the disease may have prevented the homicide. Much of the following section is concerned with an exploration of how that better control could have been achieved.

Although academic debates are trivial in relation to matters of life and death, this finding ought also to put paid to any suggestion that delusions are not important in the violence of the mentally ill (Appelbaum *et al.*, 2000, and see discussion in Chapter 2).

## The value of structured clinical assessment of violence risk (SCAVR)

Many of these Inquiries, and others before them, called for the introduction of better risk assessment procedures. Most English hospitals have some form of clinical risk assessment in place but most do not have a true, structured clinical assessment such as the HCR20. The most basic approach involves ticking boxes relating to a patient's history, and it may offer a false sense of security. An effective system requires systematic consideration of past history, present state, and future placement and stressors.

Many of the study cases reinforce the call for better risk assessment and management. There was a sense in a minority of these cases that the team had no awareness of the level of risk they were dealing with. After the event clinicians said the risk had been low, even when indications of increased risk were obvious to an Inquiry and were reflected in a structured assessment.

In the world of research much of the debate about violence risk assessment focuses on the accuracy of prediction but these cases reveal a more basic problem. Some teams were unable to formulate, describe, or communicate an assessment of violence risk. Such an assessment is multifaceted and ought to include consideration of the type of violence, the likely victims, exacerbating and alleviating factors, and the duration and immediacy of any risk. Instead, assessments were often absent. When attempted, sometimes after the event, assessments were limited to 'low' or 'high', and they were often wrong even in their own simple terms. Unstructured clinical risk assessment allows for a fair degree of latitude but there have to be some standards; referring to a high risk as a low one seems a reasonable place to draw the initial line in the sand.

The inescapable conclusion from some of these cases was that when discussing violence risk, the professionals involved literally did not know what they were talking about. There is no implied criticism of the individuals, as they had had no proper training. More than ten years after the Ritchie report, and the numerous calls for better risk assessment that followed it, this situation is hard to defend. The first step in improving risk management is to develop an agreed way of describing risk. Until there is a common language, it is impossible to make much progress.

## Recommendations

- Mental health teams need to adopt a common way of formulating, describing and communicating violence risk.
- All mental health teams should have access to a structured clinical assessment of violence risk and should incorporate its findings into the care management of patients with a history of violence.

## Compliance and compulsory treatment in the community

Lack of awareness of risk was the most worrying problem in these cases, but a commoner one was the team's inability to manage known violence risks. Risk assessment is of little value without the means to manage that risk. Non-compliance with medication was a major problem and it featured in most of the Inquiry reports. The reports contained a range of suggestions for addressing the issue, including compliance therapy, motivational interviewing, better involvement of carers and relatives, use of restriction orders to deal with previous violent offending, and better monitoring. They are all good suggestions, and most services use these strategies to a greater or lesser degree.

However, when the cases are considered together, these suggestions appear inadequate. The sample was defined by the presence of serious mental illness and previous violence, but many of these cases also had a lack of insight, accompanied by negative and hostile attitudes to services and to authority in general. Some patients had criminal or antisocial attitudes that were well entrenched before the onset of mental illness. Compliance was a problem in 23 of these 25 cases, and many of these patients were never going to comply voluntarily with medication. The task of persuasion in such patients is likely to be time-consuming, difficult, and unsuccessful, particularly because the aim is compliance with medication over many years. It is reasonable to expect a team to sustain a high level of input to ensure compliance over a brief period, but that effort cannot be sustained indefinitely. There are also resource implications. Should teams divert most of their resources to problems they probably cannot solve?

The Mental Health Act 1983 in England and Wales has no community treat-ment order or equivalent of mandated community treatment for civil patients. The only possibility for enforcing treatment in the community is in patients convicted of serious offences, who can be made the subject of a Hospital Order with restrictions, which allows for a prolonged period of conditional discharge subject to a range of conditions. In other patients there is no way of enforcing compliance in the community, a problem that has created 'revolving door patients'. This term has been applied to chronically mentally ill patients who are non-compliant in the community. They lose insight and relapse, leading to a brief admission, stabilization on medication, and discharge to a further repeti-tion of the cycle.

In these circumstances, a lot of attention focuses on when to intervene and admit the deteriorating, non-compliant patient. Several Inquiries have debated this issue, and it is common for them to argue that there should have been earlier detention. The Falling Shadow Inquiry expended enormous energy on establishing that the vagueness of mental health law allowed for detention without the necessity of waiting for an obvious relapse. Other Inquiries have reached the same conclusion, but such early intervention is rarely seen in practice and clinicians either do not accept the extent of their powers or are reluctant to use them.

Part of the problem is the futility of detention when it is just another turn of the revolving door, rather than the beginning of long-term, effective treatment. The histories of many of these patients are peppered with brief admissions, and it is unrealistic so suppose the answer is to be found in yet another admission. Schizophrenia is a chronic relapsing condition and it follows that effective compulsory treatment needs to be administered on a long-term basis. The lack of such powers has a wider detrimental effect on services by involving them in pointless, repetitive activity. Many of the homicide cases involved services struggling with difficult and dangerous patients, often with clear and well-argued reasons for refusing medication in the community. Services cannot manage such patients safely using persuasion alone and they need proper legal powers, with appropriate safeguards, to enforce compliance with treatment.

Added force is given to the case for compulsory powers by the fact that their absence has been mentioned so many times in homicide Inquiries. Case 3 above is an ideal example. The Inquiry was thorough and identified only minor issues relating to the patient's care but came to the firm conclusion that the case could only have been managed safely if there had been the power to impose treatment in the community. It is a truism of risk management that risks become less acceptable once attention has been drawn to them. The Inquiry report on Case 3 was published in 1999 and, given the stated priority of reducing violence risk, urgent consideration should be given to introducing some form of compulsory treatment in the community.

Case 3 suggests that any such change in the law would have wide ramifications. A new law could have been used in that case to good effect but the impact on other cases may have been even greater. Case 3 was an example of a team doing everything possible within existing law to measure and manage violence risk. In several other cases there was a failure to address known risks of violence, deriving in part from a sense that nothing could be done about it.

### Recommendation

◆ There is a need for legal powers to allow compulsory treatment in the community of patients with a serious mental illness and a history of violence and non-compliance.

## Drug and alcohol misuse: dual diagnosis

In all but two of the sample cases there were known problems of drug and/or alcohol misuse. The case descriptions give some indication of the importance of intoxication as a precipitating factor for violent behaviour, and in that respect the mentally ill are like other members of the community.

While there is no doubting the importance of substance misuse, the problem does not lend itself to simple solutions. There is a vast criminological literature on alcohol, drugs, and violence, and the only simple message to emerge is that the links are complicated. Apart from the direct effects of intoxication and the social decline that may result from spending money on substances rather than on life's necessities, there is a social dimension. Heavy drinking or drug use often takes place in a social environment where violence is not only acceptable but a preferred method of resolving conflict. As Case 24 illustrates, the mentally ill are not isolated from that world. Leaving aside complex questions concerning the possible effects of (treated) schizophrenia in leading to paranoid thoughts, impulsive aggression and violence, the violence in this case originated in the pub and involved the active participation and of others in whom there was no question of mental illness.

Cases such as these show the complexity of the issues facing mental health teams attempting to address the risk of violence. It is obviously right for mental health teams to respect the family and cultural background and beliefs of patients, but there is a dilemma when that background includes heavy drinking and use of illicit drugs, in a subculture that condones violence in many situations. Cannabis poses similar difficulties, with the added complication of its direct role in exacerbating psychotic symptoms.

The common response of Inquiries to substance misuse problems is to recommend the greater involvement of substance misuse services, or the setting up of specialist Dual Diagnosis teams. It is hard to disagree with this advice but it has far-reaching implications, given the frequency of the problem. The immediate question is therefore one of determining priorities.

In this respect it is useful to look at the way in which substance misuse figures in risk assessment schemes such as the HCR20. It is taken into account alongside other risk factors, both as a Historical indicator of risk, and as a Risk Management item, 'Exposure to Destabilizers'. It may also be scored under the Risk Management heading of 'Stress' if substance abuse contributes directly or indirectly to the stresses facing a patient in the community. These include the social and financial stresses that may flow from substance use. In this way, the problem of substance misuse is assessed within the wider context of the patient's life and the overall violence risk.

Substance misuse in the context of serious mental illness and violence may greatly increase risk, yet there is little sign within any of these cases of it being considered as an indication for use of compulsory powers. In Case 25 above it seems surprising that a restricted patient with a disordered mental state was known to be using cannabis over a long period. The 1983 Act does not allow detention for substance use alone, but drug use may be an important indicator of the nature and extent of a mental illness, and of the associated risks to others, so it should be included in any assessment for possible detention.

## Recommendations

◆ Substance misuse problems in patients with severe mental illness and a risk of violence should be assessed and managed within a structured clinical risk management plan. Proper consideration should always be given to the possibility of using the Mental Health Act in such patients.

◆ In patients subject to a restriction order there should always be consideration of setting conditions relating to abstinence from drugs or alcohol and the standard procedure should be immediate recall if that condition is breached.

## Early intervention and setting limits

This issue overlaps with others, particularly non-compliance and compulsion, but it deserves emphasis. In at least seven of these cases, including Cases 8, 19, and 25, one of whom was a conditionally discharged restricted patient, there was a strong case for earlier intervention. The teams knew there was a problem; they worried about it; but they did not know where to draw the line when there was deteriorating behaviour, non-compliance, or drug misuse. The problem goes beyond limits on legal powers, as there was no proper consideration of those limits.

It has become common for care-planning meetings to list warning signs and indicators of relapse but the missing ingredient was intervention. One can only speculate as to the reasons. In some cases it may be over-familiarity. The cannabis smoker with the abnormal mental state had been like that for a long time. Forensic services may have become too accustomed to dealing with a high level of risk, forgetting that in high-risk cases in the community intervention should come earlier rather than later. In other cases it may be lack of confidence in the benefits of treatment.

## Recommendations

◆ There should be early intervention when there are signs of deterioration or risky behaviours in patients with a history of violence. This principle should rarely if ever be ignored, even when a patient is well known to the service. If in doubt, the team should err on the side of caution.

◆ When dealing with patients with a history of violence and serious mental illness, care-planning meetings should set clear, operational criteria for intervention. These criteria should be communicated to, and when possible agreed with, patients and carers so they have realistic expectations.

## Forensic and general psychiatry services

Forensic services were not directly involved in most of these cases at the time of the homicide and there were worrying aspects to those cases in which they did have responsibility. There did not appear to be any systematic basis for whether patients were managed by one or the other service. The decision did not appear to be based on risk, which would be the obvious criterion. Case 2 was an exception, where there had been a recent opinion from a forensic psychiatrist that greatly strengthened the position of the team at the Inquiry.

### Recommendations

- The basis for referral of cases between general and forensic teams should be a structured clinical assessment of violence risk.
- A forensic opinion should be sought in respect of those patients with the highest level of violence risk.
- Forensic teams should manage patients in the community with a higher level of supervision than the general team can provide. They should intervene earlier when there is deterioration, because of the higher background risk of violence.

## Diagnosis and the medical model

Diagnosis is important in risk management because the identification of a mental illness implies the availability of an effective treatment. Diagnosis is less important in the assessment of violence risk and is correctly considered as just one of many factors.

In some of these cases teams expended a lot of time and effort on the question of the correct diagnosis, while failing to recognize the violence risks involved. If there is an adequate risk management plan in place, based on a provisional diagnosis, a definitive label can safely wait.

There were particular problems over the diagnosis of drug-induced psychosis, which seemed to be approached with an emphasis on voluntary intoxication, and insufficient recognition that it is a psychosis with the same potential for disaster as in schizophrenia. As many if not most patients with schizophrenia use drugs, usually to the detriment of their mental state, the distinction between schizophrenia and drug-induced psychosis is often impossible and of little practical importance.

Personality disorder also presented difficulties, as it was too often seen as precluding the need for a full assessment of risk, and sometimes as a reason for not offering a full treatment package. This leaves services vulnerable when schizophrenia later proves to be the correct diagnosis.

### Recommendations

- Violence risk assessment should be undertaken early in a patient's contact with services. It will always be subject to revision as new information emerges but it should never depend on the presence of a specific diagnosis alone.

◆ The diagnosis of drug-induced psychosis should be discouraged or abandoned.

## Involvement of carers

This is a complex issue, as illustrated by those cases in which carers opposed necessary intervention or participated in antisocial behaviour that made violence more likely. Notwithstanding these difficulties, there was a worrying lack of involvement of carers in some cases, and in others their clearly expressed concerns about violence were ignored. This is a particularly serious failing given that carers or relatives are most exposed to violence risk.

### Recommendations

◆ Concern about violence risk should be shared openly with patients and with carers whenever possible, supported by copies of care plans and other relevant documents.

◆ The assessment of violence risk should be thoroughly reviewed whenever the carer appears more worried than the team.

## The inevitability of violence

The focus of this chapter, and of the whole book, is on improving care as a means to prevent violence but some of these cases demonstrate that serious violence cannot always be predicted or prevented. This is particularly the case when the violence is coincident with the mental illness rather than a consequence of it. Any review of Inquiry reports is bound to expose the unfairness of some comments made with the benefit of hindsight. Not all violence by the mentally ill can be prevented, and services need support and encouragement in acknowledgment of that unfortunate fact.

### Recommendation

◆ An effective strategy for managing serious violence by patients needs to recognize that it is sometimes inevitable, and that strategy should offer support to staff as well as reassurance to the public.

## Types of violence in schizophrenia

The range of cases encountered in this study raises the question of how to classify acts that are unified by their occurrence in mental illness but in other respects have little in common.

Some authors make a case for there being two types of violence in schizophrenia (Steinert *et al.*, 1998; Gje *et al.*, 2003). Mullen (2006, in press) summarizes Type 1 patients as having insignificant histories of conduct disorder or adult delinquency, with a first violent offence after the onset of the illness. They are likely to have delusional systems that relate directly to their violence, they 'almost always attack a carer or acquaintance, and … look like patients'. Type 2 violence occurs in patients with a history of conduct disorder, substance mis-use, and offending (both violent and non-violent) predating the onset of the mental illness. The clinical picture is usually disorganized, chaotic, and impulsive. They commit violence in both domestic and non-domestic settings and they 'look like criminals'. Mullen suggests that Type 2 patients account for the majority of violence in schizophrenia, but Type 1 may be over-represented among homicide offenders.

The good thing about this approach is the attempt to distinguish different types and dimensions of violence. But because there are so many dimensions—the summary above includes historical, developmental, social, and illness characteristics—it is unlikely that cases will fit neatly into two categories. The Type 1 and Type 2 terminology has been taken straight from physical medicine where it has been applied to diseases such as diabetes. Even in diabetes there may be overlap between the two groups, and that problem is bound to be greater in the more nebulous world of violence and psychosis.

As an aside, one has to wonder why psychiatry is so obsessed with dubious classification systems while turning a deaf ear to the real message to be taken from the treatment of diabetes: when treating a life-long disease, it is a serious mistake to stop medication that is keeping the patient well.

Turning back to the classification of violence, it is better to describe it with reference to these various dimensions rather than to shoehorn cases into boxes that do not really fit. Some previous research supports this view. Laajasalo and Hakkanen (2001) looked at all 109 Finnish homicide offenders in the period from 1983 to 2002 and compared those whose offending began early, before the onset of mental illness, and late. There were few differences between the groups. Patients in the late onset group were more likely to have victimized a relative, possibly because the early onset group were more likely to have alienated family and to have less contact with them.

In the present study, any attempt to divide the patients into early- or late-starting offenders would have been misleading. Two archetypal killings of a stranger (Cases 8 and 17) involved patients who were not antisocial before the onset of their illness. Yet once they became ill their behaviour was chaotic, irresponsible, and antisocial almost all the time—except when they were taking medication. Any system of classification into Types 1 or 2 is bound to lead to serious errors in which patients of this type are written off as having serious conduct and behaviour problems independent of their mental illness.

The reality in these cases was that mental illness made them that way. It is only a small step from deciding that a patient looks like a criminal, to deciding he should be in prison rather than in the clinic.

The message is that schizophrenia affects all aspects of personality functioning. Severe forms of the disease can mimic many of the features of psychopathy, including lack of empathy, emotional coldness, impulsivity, irresponsibility, and lack of remorse. On present state alone, it becomes virtually impossible to distinguish those who had psychopathic features then became mentally ill, from those who developed psychopathic features after the onset of the illness. Robert Hare's pragmatic solution to this problem is to rate the Psychopathy Checklist according to the features present, irrespective of their origins, because psychopathy correlates with violence risk in any event.

Hare's advice is good for the assessment of violence risk but treatment is a different matter, and here the distinction becomes crucial. Is this a case in which effective treatment will dramatically reduce the violence risk, or will it make little difference? If in doubt, all the odds favour assertive treatment because the consequences of a false positive error (giving medication to a patient whose main problem is a severe personality disorder) are less serious than the consequences of the false negative error (omitting treatment that would greatly reduce violence risk). Either way, a proper formulation of the case requires a developmental history in addition to an assessment of current mental state.

## Conclusions

The point of this chapter, along with Chapter 3, is to illustrate the enormous gap between the concerns of researchers, and the reality of risk management in clinical practice. The homicide reports and Inquiries have been quoted at some length to demonstrate the extent to which the problems they identify differ from the concerns of researchers. In a small number of cases violence seems to come out of the blue, or has no apparent link to the mental illness, but most concern offences in which psychotic symptoms were the main or only motivation, and in which the indicators of risk were all too obvious.

In the real world, clinicians do not usually struggle with the theoretical limits of risk assessment and technology. In most cases they make no attempt to use that technology because they are unaware or untrained. Many existing risk assessments are simple, one-dimensional affairs that do not assist management. Even when the risk assessment is good, it is not linked to a proper risk management plan. Clinicians lack the power to enforce risk management in the community, and they seem reluctant to use the powers they have. Risk assessment is too often mixed up with diagnostic issues yet, paradoxically, there is a reluctance to intervene in chronic schizophrenia even when there is a disturbed mental state and a history of previous violence and present drug misuse.

The assumption throughout this chapter is that we are considering the tip of the iceberg or, to be precise, the tips of several icebergs. If not, then these comments may be unfair and reflect the scientific error of looking only at cases in which the outcome was bad. Perhaps these are the anomalies, and the rest of mental health care proceeds in an orderly, rational, and safe manner. If so, this book is pointless and unnecessary. Anomaly or iceberg? Readers familiar with mental health services are invited to decide for themselves.

Chapter 8

# Conclusions: on good treatment and bad attitudes

## On the meaning of life ...

So what is it all about then, this business of mental health care and violence? And what have we learned?

This final chapter begins with a summary of the principles of violence risk management. It is only a summary; earlier chapters explored the surrounding arguments, so the debate will not be repeated here. Instead, I list 10 principles. I could have called them commandments but we are, or aspire to be, scientists.

The second part of the chapter is where the philosophy comes in. It goes beyond the mechanics of risk management to consider why mental health services sometimes get it wrong. There is more to this matter than technical failures, hence the concern with meaning and attitudes.

The third section considers ethics and the legal framework within which services operate, and the final section deals with the organizational and managerial framework within which we operate. While most of this book is addressed directly to clinicians, it is appropriate to end with a reminder that big improvements in clinical risk management will require full organizational support.

## Ten principles of violence risk management

1. *Violence is your business.* Violence is an important complication of schizophrenia—and of some other mental disorders, but principles have to be pithy. Schizophrenia is found in 1% of the general population, and in 5% of people in the UK who are charged with homicide. If you work in mental health, you cannot ignore the risk of violence.

2. *There is no alternative to violence risk management.* Do not be seduced by the suggestion that a capacity test is a viable alternative. If you detain patients on the grounds of risk to others you already assess violence risk, and there is an unanswerable case for doing it better.

3. *Good violence risk management is good for patients.* Risk management is not about locking up patients. The goal is optimum treatment supported by an explicit, transparent plan for managing all the risks associated with their illness, including the risk of violence. It is never in a patient's best interest to allow him to commit an act of serious violence. In order to reduce the chances of that outcome, we have a duty to use the best risk management technology.

4. *Hope for the best but plan for the worst.* Optimism has its place but health services need to consider the possibility of a negative outcome, and to make reasonable contingency plans. If a patient has been violent before he will probably be violent again and crossed fingers are not an adequate response.

   Under the same heading I would also include a warning against using the optimist's diagnosis of drug-induced psychosis whenever violence is involved. The label is optimistic because it assumes the patient may avoid drugs in the future, and it assumes he will not become psychotic if he avoids drugs. In many cases time will prove both assumptions wrong. Better to play safe and treat it as schizophrenia, which is a less serious mistake to make.

5. *Prediction is impossible but prevention can be easy.* An overemphasis on the problem of prediction has damaged the cause of violence risk management. We are not fortune-tellers but we are risk managers, just like professionals in any other branch of medicine. Homicide Inquiries show that following basic policies and procedures would often have prevented serious violence. Compliance with the correct medication greatly reduces the risk of violence in schizophrenia.

6. *Not all violent acts are equal.* The killing of another person for psychotic motives is the worst possible negative outcome in the treatment of serious mental illness. Prevention is not always possible but it must be a priority for services, and it is of the highest priority when there is a history of psychotic violence. In such circumstances treatment and compliance become matters of concern to others, outside the doctor–patient relationship. Violence that is incidental to the mental illness must be taken into account in risk management but it places different obligations on the service. We need to have realistic expectations in such circumstances and we need to educate politicians. If mental health services treat violent people it should be no surprise that some continue to behave violently for reasons unconnected with their illness or treatment.

7. *Standardized assessments help clinicians but do not replace them.* Actuarial methods are perfect for planners and managers but they have limited value

for clinicians dealing with individuals. It is never acceptable to use an actuarial assessment alone as a substitute for a full clinical assessment of an individual patient. On the other hand, the additional use of actuarial assessments will improve many clinical assessments and is essential in sex offenders and those with personality disorders. The evidence in favour of structured clinical assessment is overwhelming. The assessment should include consideration of the future, in terms of possible negative outcomes and plans for managing risks. The central role of clinical discretion means there is no absolute certainty, so team working and the use of second opinions are important safeguards. A risk shared is a risk halved, as the old saying almost goes.

8. *Aspire to the best but give what you can afford.* The correct order of events is to decide on the optimum safe management of a case, then to worry about how and whether it is possible to provide that treatment. Reasons for any shortfall must be documented but in the real world of competing demands, patients will not always get everything they need. The serious error is to tailor the recommendation to fit what is available ('there is no bed so the patient does not need admission'). This approach is illogical, unethical, and counter-productive because it conceals shortcomings in service provision.

9. *Write it down.* A risk assessment does not exist until it is committed to paper. The extent of what needs to be written down depends on the nature of the service, the extent of the risk, and the history of violence. Once a risk has been recorded, the actions to address that risk must be recorded alongside it. It makes no sense to note the risk without noting the action to be taken, even if there is no definitive solution.

10. *When in doubt, treat.* The next section, on philosophy, will develop further the theme of reluctance to treat. The science is unambiguous. In schizophrenia or other serious mental illness the balance of risks favours treatment. Once a risk of violence is introduced to the equation, the weight of evidence in favour of assertive treatment is overwhelming. As a consequence it is easier to defend a decision to treat, even if the outcome is negative. The most risky decision is to deny treatment or to turn a patient away.

Do not be deterred from attempting treatment by concern that a Tribunal will not support compulsion. If you treat psychotic patients with a history of violence and the law is not holding you back some of the time, you are probably not trying hard enough.

## Attitude problems

When reading homicide Inquiries, it soon becomes obvious that many involve not technical or organizational failures but problems of attitude. Too many people working in mental health services lack Attitude, and those who have it are often embarrassed about it. Risks are recognized, but there is a reluctance to intervene. Professionals emphasize the rights of the violent patient to refuse treatment, at the expense of the rights of others to be protected. Doctors underestimate their legal powers to detain and treat patients. The default position is to do nothing.

Yet the point of mental health services is to deliver treatment. Why do so many Inquiries reveal a lack of assertiveness on the part of services? Why do we lack confidence in the value of treatment?

## I blame RD Laing

RD Laing, father of the antipsychiatry movement in the 1960s, has a lot to answer for. A charismatic man with a talent for self-promotion, his useful contributions to the treatment of schizophrenia would fit on the back of a non-existent postage stamp but his books were bestsellers and they remain in print. Laing (1970) popularized the notion that the family and society cause schizophrenia and psychiatrists, as agents of control for an oppressive state, make it worse with their poisonous drugs: a hippy version of Foucault, with psychoanalysis thrown in to add credibility.

Laing's scientific credibility is non-existent and his ideas have been attacked on other grounds, mainly as a distasteful attempt to blame the patient or the family for being ill (he was, after all, a doctor). But if his scientific impact was negligible, his cultural impact was massive and his true legacy is a lingering stench attached to mental health care. Stigma associated with mental illness has a much longer history but Laing can be blamed for—or credited with, depending on your ideology—adding to the stigma associated with treatment. He promoted the belief that psychiatric treatment is a bad thing, that patients need protecting from it, and that they are better left to their own devices.

This is nonsense, but Laing was entitled to his opinion. We live in a free society. In fact, we live in an adversarial society, where consensus often emerges from a struggle between conflicting values. Extremes of opinion keep professions in check and remind us of our powers and responsibilities. RD Laing should not be criticized for being good at promoting his ideas, even if they were wrong.

Instead, the fault lies with those in mental health to whom Laing should provide a counterbalance. Dissect most psychiatrists and at the heart you find a pellet of antipsychiatry, about the size of a rabbit dropping, with 'Laing' inscribed on it. Antipsychiatry permeated the profession so thoroughly that we have all become, to an extent, antipsychiatrists.

Ambivalence about our work defines psychiatry's difference from other medical specialties. Cardiac surgeons fight for new technology. Renal physicians battle for better transplant facilities. Cancer specialists campaign for more supplies of the latest, eye-wateringly expensive drug. And psychiatrists campaign for human rights.

Not that there is anything wrong with campaigning for human rights. Only that psychiatrists have no training or skills in the area, and plenty of people do it better. Meanwhile, if the doctors are manning the barricades to ensure their own patients are protected from them, who is left to campaign for more and better mental health care? In the UK, the task has fallen to voluntary groups such as the Zito Trust or Sane and, ironically, the Government. It is at least arguable that the main service improvements in relation to violence and mental health care have come about despite the profession, rather than as a result of it. Go figure.

## Towards a better service

The first step in improving risk management is to recognize that the prevention of violence is a central task of mental health services. Once a mental disorder is associated with violence and a risk to others, the risk–benefit scales tilt firmly in favour of intervention. No reticence or apology is necessary. The mistake of treating too early will always be more acceptable than the potential disaster of treating too late.

In the real world, of course, there are many obstacles. If an assertive approach becomes insensitive it jeopardizes relationships with patients or carers, although anecdotal evidence suggests carers would welcome greater involvement in more assertive care. The key lies in working with families and carers, who are often most concerned about violence risk.

Services should be explicit about the risks of violence from the start. Care planning meetings in patients with a history of violence should include plans for dealing with relapse and increased risk. The plans should be agreed with patient and carer whenever possible, with copies to take away. It is much easier to intervene early when patient and carer have been given clear expectations that this is what will happen in case of relapse or deterioration.

## Getting people to do what they don't want to do: the ethics of caring for violent patients

Beyond the mechanics of individual care, the profession needs to engage in more open ethical debates about violence. When is it ethically acceptable to enforce compliance in a patient who is stable but has been violent before and will probably become violent again if he relapses? Individual practitioners make such decisions all the time, but there is little general debate. In the same vein, what should services do about violent patients who misuse illicit drugs? Should we take a different attitude to cannabis use in violent patients?

The conventional interpretation of ethics in relation to mental health is a preoccupation with the autonomy of the patient, so acres of print have been devoted to arguments for mental capacity as the sole arbiter for compulsory treatment. It is easy for these arguments to take on a rather smug quality, as we are all in favour of autonomy and choice. Meanwhile, we operate in a real world where many decisions hinge on risk. We need a more difficult ethical debate about the extent to which the risk of violence, based on a past history, justifies interference with patient autonomy. Mental health teams struggle with decisions of this type every day, and they need to be supported by open discussion and debate within the profession. Without such a debate, a lack of confidence will continue to jeopardize assertive approaches to treatment.

To understand why a lack of confidence is such a problem, it is helpful to return to the question posed at the start of the chapter: what is it all about? We can probably agree that services are 'about' providing treatment, but the question is more interesting and more difficult when applied to the management of violence risk. How does the role of the service change when patients are more difficult and less co-operative?

Essentially, the job of the psychiatrist and the service is to get patients to do things they do not want to do. There is a bit more to it, but the task of begging, persuading, and sometimes compelling reluctant compliance lies at the heart of mental health care when managing violence risk. The ethics of this approach are complicated in a service that values autonomy and choice, but they are not impossible. Addictions services work with reluctant clients all the time. They recognize the importance of persuasion and have made it an explicit and central part of their ethos through motivational interviewing (Miller and Rollnick, 1992). General mental health services could benefit from a similar approach, both in developing better techniques but also in adopting the attitude or mindset. Respect for autonomy is important, but part of the job is getting people to do things they would not otherwise do. It follows that one measure of success for the service is how well it manages to treat people whose first, free choice would be to stay away.

Critics will mutter about paternalism, but there are worse things than fathers. Relations and carers are usually allies in the task of persuasion, so it is important to involve them fully and to understand their concerns. Ethical questions arise from potential conflicts between obligations to the family/carer and to the individual patient. However, like most ethical dilemmas, it is much easier to resolve when violence risk is involved. In case of doubt the best advice is to share information with the family. It would be good to see these issues more widely debated within the profession. Meanwhile, services should develop policies for the guidance and protection of staff.

## Support for staff

The value of recognizing persuasion and coercion as important parts of the job is that we can confront the problems involved. Some of those problems are ethical but others are psychological. The task of getting people to do things they do not want to do is difficult, demanding, and draining. It involves repeatedly sitting across a table from a patient and telling him you do not agree with the request to reduce medication—and he should lay off the cannabis/crack/alcohol, and stop hanging with undesirables. Usually the patient is socially and economically disadvantaged, possibly from an ethnic minority, and it is easy to start feeling like the agent of social control that Laing warned us about. After a few years of this, staff may yearn to deal with co-operative and grateful patients who bring presents at Christmas—and they may start to say yes when the answer should be no.

Some mental health disasters arise because of a failure to set proper limits in patients who have been known to services for a long time (see Chapter 7). Part of the problem is complacency borne out of familiarity, but there is also a tendency to grow jaded by the conflict. It is hard work, saying no all the time. Services need to address these issues in support for frontline staff, and we need to be explicit about this aspect of mental health work. There is conflict as well as consensus, and we should feel comfortable with both. Too much published work on the ethics of mental health focuses on the human rights of the patient and leaves this aspect of our work feeling like a grubby, marginal activity rather than the mainstay of violence risk management.

## Mental health law

It may seem strange to be getting around to the law at this late stage in the book but it is no accident, for several reasons. The law varies between countries and changes with time, whereas the principles of violence risk management are constant. The law and clinical practice may intersect but they are separate, with their own value systems. Risk management has suffered from an overemphasis on the law and legal concepts, to the detriment of clinical initiatives.

All medical disciplines manage clinical risk, but only in psychiatry is there such an emphasis on the legal aspects. As a result, clinicians in mental health have been too ready to leave it to the law, whereas the correct sequence of events is:

1. Clinicians formulate optimum risk management plans.
2. Clinicians look to the law to see what it allows them to do.
3. Clinicians modify plans as necessary then do what they can.
4. Clinicians advise on and request changes in the law when prevents them from doing their job.

Of course, they may not get the changes they ask for because other principles and parties are involved and the law is not there for the convenience of doctors. Even so, the model is correct in its emphasis on clinicians driving the process of risk assessment and management as part of mainstream clinical practice. The law sets limits on what can be done, but it is not the driving force.

The most relevant law in relation to violence risk management concerns powers of compulsory detention or treatment. It may also allow coercive treatment within the criminal justice system. A full discussion is beyond the scope of this book, and only a brief statement of principles will be attempted.

Mental health law allows compulsory detention or treatment when certain conditions are fulfilled. There are separate statutes for people who have been convicted of an offence (criminal statutes) and for those who have not (civil statutes).

## Civil versus criminal mental health legislation

The general principle of civil mental health law is that compulsion is permissible when certain criteria are fulfilled, even if no criminal law has been broken. The criteria are related to the presence of a mental disorder and, in broad terms, risk (whether to self or others) or impaired decision-making capacity or competence. The differences between these approaches were discussed in Chapter 1. There may also be differences in whether civil detention requires the involvement of a court or Tribunal in the first instance, as in Scotland or the USA, or whether it is reviewed by a court at a later stage, as in England and Wales. The absence of any review by a court or other judicial body would be incompatible with human rights legislation.

Criminal mental health legislation comes into play to allow compulsory treatment or detention after a mentally disordered offender has been convicted. In some jurisdictions the mental disorder may also influence the criminal proceedings and lead to a verdict of not guilty by reason of insanity, or that the offender is unfit to plead or to stand trial. These complications are not important here, where the main point is that the law allows a range of sentences that are designed to allow risk management through treatment.

Two examples are the Hospital Order in England and Wales and the TBS ('Terbeschikkingstelling') order in the Netherlands.

### The Hospital Order in England and Wales

A convicted offender may be sentenced to detention in hospital as an alternative to other punishments such as prison. Although there is deprivation of liberty, there is no intended component of punishment to this sentence. Discharge from the order is at the discretion of the treating psychiatrist with no further reference to the court. The sentence is a once-and-for-all alternative to imprisonment and there is no way of reversing the decision and sending the patient from hospital to prison.

For the most serious offences a Restriction Order may be imposed, which means that the right of discharge is vested in the Home Secretary or a Tribunal. Discharge from a restricted Hospital Order is usually conditional, which allows for a prolonged period of compulsory treatment in the community.

### The TBS order in the Netherlands

The TBS order is imposed by a court on convicted violent or sexual offenders with a mental disorder who are though to present a continuing risk. The offender first serves a determinate prison sentence set by the court to reflect the nature of the offence, and is then transferred for indeterminate detention and treatment in a TBS unit until the risk has been sufficiently reduced to allow release under supervision. The interesting contrast with English legislation is the explicit element of punishment. In this respect the English law has more reciprocity than the Dutch, because it sets aside all punishment in favour of treatment.

## Risk management and the law

The law grants most powers to services in the case of patients who have broken the law, which is consistent with principles of human rights and natural justice. The problem for services is that mentally disordered offenders in many jurisdictions are less likely than other offenders to end up with a conviction, or they end up with a lesser conviction, even when they have committed violent offences. Many countries have a deliberate policy of diverting mentally disordered offenders away from the criminal justice system, which was meant to keep petty offenders out of prison and is sometimes wrongly applied to more serious offenders. There is often an additional reluctance of the police or prosecutors to proceed with prosecutions against the mentally ill. The intentions are good but can result in serious offences being overlooked by the criminal justice system, a problem highlighted by the Clunis case (see Chapter 3) and other homicide Inquiries. The result is that services are left to struggle with serious offenders, without the benefit of the additional powers that may result from conviction.

The main practical problem in the absence of a conviction for a serious offence is the inability to enforce compliance with medication after discharge, which is possible in the UK with offender-patients who have been sentenced to a Hospital Order with restrictions, but not for civil patients. The UK Government has announced plans to introduce a community treatment order that will allow compulsory treatment provided certain conditions are met, even if there has never been a conviction. Meanwhile, services continue to struggle with the problem. Many hospitals have developed arrangements with the police for joint working, so that patients are diverted to treatment when they commit minor offences but serious offences are prosecuted.

The other important development in England and Wales is the advent of Multi-Agency Public Protection Panels, which deal only with offenders but provide assistance in managing those offender patients who are not subject to a Restriction Order. See Royal College of Psychiatrists (2005) for a fuller account of Muli-Agency Public Protection Arrangements in the UK.

It should be noted that mental health legislation is not intended to deal with all the risks associated with mental disorder. In serious offences the correct disposal may be a life sentence rather than a Hospital Order, because the former assumes a wider approach to risk management beyond the purely medical. Many psychiatrists argue that an indeterminate Hospital Order is never a satisfactory disposal for an offender with psychopathic disorder alone. If the court believes the risks are high enough the correct sentence is life imprisonment, which allows for treatment as part of that sentence but does not leave the patient stranded in a psychiatric hospital if treatment is unsuccessful. On a more everyday level, probation orders with a condition of treatment involve an element of coercion while retaining flexibility.

Further consideration of the law is beyond the scope of this book but the next section concerns one of the principles underlying mental health law, that of reciprocity.

## Legal principles: reciprocity in mental health

The principle of reciprocity insists that when society curtails the freedom of a mentally disordered person, because of the mental disorder and its associated risks, there is an obligation to provide treatment for the mental disorder.

In its weakest form, this principle is enshrined in human rights legislation. Article 5 of the European convention allows for '... the lawful detention of persons of unsound mind ...,' but insists that such detention is in '... a hospital, clinic or other appropriate institution authorised for the detention of such people'. It is not acceptable to hold the mentally disordered in a prison or other place of punishment when he has not been convicted of a crime, and the use of hospital or clinic implies that some sort of care will be provided. This general principle is unlikely to provoke much argument, but there is more room for controversy when we consider the details of the care to be provided.

What about conditions for which there is no effective treatment? The extreme form of the reciprocity argument claims it is not acceptable to detain a mentally disordered person unless the mental disorder is likely to respond to treatment. This is an extension of the 'pure' ethical position outlined above. The role of the doctor is to relieve her patient's suffering, so she has no business detaining any patient for any other reason, no matter how compelling, if she has no effective treatment to offer.

Anyone familiar with the Mental Health Act 1983 in England and Wales will recognize this principle in the additional condition that must be satisfied before patients can be detained under the legal categories of psychopathic disorder or mental impairment. It is necessary to show that treatment is likely to alleviate or prevent deterioration in the mental disorder, even when detention is necessary for the safety of the patient, or for the safety of others.

While this is not a history book, a brief digression into the origins of this phrase helps to shed some light on the tensions in this area between public protection on the one hand and the rights of patients on the other. The first consideration was to protect people of low intelligence from indefinite detention in a hospital, despite risk to self or others, if the hospital could do nothing to help them. Hence, mental impairment was treated differently from mental illness or severe mental impairment, in that the diagnosis could not be used to justify detention unless the condition was treatable. This is an understandable safeguard, particularly because it was drawn up when deinstitutionalization was at an early stage. The scandals surrounding abuses in large subnormality hospitals were still emerging, and it was possible to encounter elderly women who had spent their adult life in hospital for nothing more disordered than having a baby out of wedlock.

The issues are straightforward in mental impairment but the case of psychopathic disorder is more complicated. Concern for the rights of patients was a factor, and other parts of the Act show that those who wrote it had civil liberties at the forefront of their minds. For example, the Act states explicitly that promiscuity, abnormal sexual preference, or the abuse of drugs or alcohol, are not to be regarded as mental disorders or grounds for detention.

At the same time other, less liberal, impulses were operating and many politicians argued that psychopathy should never be a reason for hospitalization. According to their view of the world, people with a personality disorder are responsible for their actions and the law should take its proper course, unhindered by psychiatrists, when psychopaths commit offences. They should be punished by being sent to prison, not sent to hospital.

In some ways, the most interesting aspect of this debate is the implicit and automatic assumption that people with a mental illness are not responsible for their actions, and I return to this issue later. For present purposes we need only note the strong opposition to any inclusion of psychopathic disorder as grounds for detention. The 1983 Act was a compromise. Doctors would be allowed to detain psychopaths in hospital, but only when they could be confident that treatment would be effective. Otherwise, the behaviour of people suffering from psychopathic disorder would be subject to all the normal legal sanctions.

The concept of effective treatment has turned out to be more ambiguous than it must have seemed at the time. I would guess that those who drew up the law imagined that treatment would take care of all the risks associated with the disorder. Instead, the Act has spawned an entire medico-legal industry of its own, to debate the meaning of 'treatment', 'ameliorate', and 'deterioration'. In response the courts have shown themselves willing to take the widest possible view of what constitutes treatment, rather than order the discharge of a dangerous patient because he is no longer treatable. In the lawyer's world, treatment may amount to nothing more than routine nursing care and residence in a hospital.

To many people, this seems like a sensible and pragmatic solution. It is fully compatible with Human Rights legislation, which makes no reference to treatment being likely to help. Parliament would surely not have handed over the care of dangerous people to psychiatrists if it anticipated that the psychiatrists would release patients who were still dangerous, simply because there was nothing more that could be done to help them. To the most extreme proponents of the reciprocity principle, however, this is an abuse of psychiatry; they argue that patients should not be detained in hospital if there is no effective treatment for their condition.

Such a narrow, literal interpretation of the concept of reciprocity is confused and illogical. In the simpler world of physical medicine, doctors have always been prepared to sanction the detention of patients with infectious diseases, in order to protect others from infection. It would be bizarre to argue they should do so only when the disease is treatable. The main concern is about diseases that are not easy to treat, when control of carriers is one of the few methods of preventing an epidemic. Psychiatrists detain a small number of dangerous patients because they are dangerous, and only because they are dangerous. We should not need to pretend that we are detaining them for their own direct benefit.

Still, we should not discard reciprocity completely. It is a more useful concept at the level of society rather than the individual. Every mentally disordered offender who is sentenced to treatment rather than punishment is engaged in a system of reciprocity. Under the law in England and Wales, a mentally disordered person may commit the most serious of crimes and yet not spend a day in prison, when a similar crime in a man without a mental disorder would carry a sentence of many years, if not life. The reciprocal expectation in return for this benefit to the individual is that the patient will accept restrictions on his liberty for as long as necessary, and that he will cooperate in his future treatment. There is also an expectation on mental health services that such treatment will give priority to minimizing the risk of re-offending. In a minority of cases, this will mean that an individual patient spends a long time in hospital because treatment does not bring the risk under control, but most pass through the system relatively quickly and have the benefit of better treatment than would be available in prison.

## Reciprocity and Nimby-ism

*NIMBY*: Not In My Back Yard. Mildly derogatory term applied to those who oppose socially desirable development because of its direct impact on them or on their property.

In discussing this issue with various audiences, it became apparent that most clinicians worry less about the principle of detaining untreatable patients, which they do routinely in the case of treatment-refractory mental illnesses, than they worry about the practicalities. They do not want the untreatable patients on their ward. Mental health services do not want their hospitals to be filled with patients who will not get better, and who may "block" beds for years. I agree, but see no reason for a law when good management is enough.

On one level this is an example of a well-established medical phenomenon. Doctors, when reluctant to do something, get together and decide that nothing can be done. But there are serious, underlying issues. The desire to maintain a flow of patients through a service is good medical management, and all sorts of problems develop in long-stay, Cinderella services. It is a sad reflection on the state of the profession that clinicians do not have the confidence to stand up and assert their requirements for running a safe and effective service, feeling instead that they have to present their concerns in moral, ethical, or legal terms.

Poor management and a reluctance to acknowledge the problem have compounded the problem of long stay patients. High secure hospitals in England and Wales contain a significant but unknown number of patients whose prospects of ever being discharged are slim. The same is probably true of medium secure units. The reasons have nothing to do with a failure to treat these patients assertively. There is simply no effective treatment in this tiny minority, and their history of serious offending means the stakes are unacceptably high.

It is tempting to avoid the issue by saying that one should not start from here, and I would argue that one should never recommend an indefinite Hospital Order for a patient with psychopathic disorder. But, however careful we are about such decisions, any inpatient service dealing with violence risk is bound to end up with some long-stay patients. Services need to make proper plans for them, and there is no justification for the failure to do so.

Holland has adopted a more rational and pragmatic approach. Its TBS system holds patients on the equivalent of indefinite, restricted Hospital Orders. All patients receive at least 5 years of attempts at active therapy but, if there has been no progress in that time, there is a shift of emphasis to maximizing quality of life within a secure setting. About 20% of all patients within the TBS system are designated in this way, and the service is managed to meet their needs.

If the UK is to have a better system of risk assessment and management within mental health services, it will need to adopt a similar approach. Services should be designed to meet a patient's needs, informed by a rational assessment of risk. It is pointless to introduce tools for better risk assessment, if their use is distorted by clinicians' fears that if they identify risks, they will be left to struggle with them in inappropriate settings with inadequate resources. On that note, we move on to consider the organizational framework within which risk is managed.

## Risk and managers: safer organizations

The law provides a context for clinical risk management but for most clinicians the immediate constraint is the service within which they work. There are limits to what individuals can achieve within a system that is increasingly governed by policies and guidelines, where improvements in individual practice are likely to be effective only if they are supported by institutional change. Relatively little attention has been paid to the organizational aspects of risk management, perhaps because one of the ways in which doctors and lawyers are united is in a tendency to focus on the individual. So when things go wrong, the subsequent Inquiry is more likely to concentrate on individual rather than organizational deficiencies.

This is a short-sited view, and it is no accident that the National Confidential Inquiry into Homicides and Suicides by Psychiatric Patients in the UK chose the title 'Safer Services' for its report. The Confidential Inquiry was meant to improve upon the methods of the Homicide Inquiries, and begins by taking a wider view of responsibility. If clinicians are to modify their practice to reduce risk effectively, they will require the involvement and support of the institutions in which they practice.

Organizations vary in their approach to safety and risk management, just as they vary in the emphasis they place on other aspects of quality, such as increasing market share or making a profit. A multinational retailer would not expect to improve its performance simply by exhorting the sales force to try harder, and safety also requires a broader, institutional strategy.

Tidmarsh (1997) made this point using the real-life example of an airliner whose pilot died at the controls. The plane landed safely with all passengers, not through good luck but because the airline had an effective safety culture. Problems had been anticipated, and contingency planning minimized the impact when a serious problem occurred.

The principle is expanded in a growing literature on High Reliability Organizations (HROs). These are organizations that must protect themselves against rare but catastrophic events. For example, nuclear aircraft carriers or the nuclear power industry cannot afford to have accidents, because of the catastrophic consequences. It would be reckless and even absurd for such organizations to rely only on individual effort, and the key to their success lies in the systems they have set up to guard against human error. Think of Homer Simpson's performance at the Springfield nuclear plant if you remain unconvinced of this point.

Unlike nuclear plants, hospitals do not count as HROs because of their high rate of errors, and it is unrealistic to think that psychiatric services can be transformed overnight. But if we are serious about giving priority to risk, we can learn from the principles by which HROs succeed.

## Principles of managing High Reliability Organizations

A study of HROs, including nuclear aircraft carriers, air traffic control, nuclear power generation, and hostage negotiation, identified five principles of successful management (Weick and Sutcliffe, 2001):

1. Preoccupation with failure.
2. Reluctance to simplify.
3. Sensitivity to operations.
4. Commitment to resilience.
5. Deference to expertise.

## Preoccupation with failure

The safest organizations spend a lot of time worrying about disasters that never happen. They recognize that things do go wrong, and they make contingency plans to deal with problems.

This is probably the main weakness of risk management in generic mental health services, which are based on the assumption that things will probably turn out all right in the end. Health workers are inclined to be professionally optimistic, partly in order to motivate and encourage patients and their families. Optimism is a useful therapeutic tool but not to be confused with a realistic assessment of risk. Psychiatry deals mainly with relapsing, chronic conditions, particularly in mentally disordered offenders, and it is unreasonable to cross one's fingers and hope for the best.

The main element of our safety culture in this respect is the Care Programme Approach (CPA), with its emphasis on care plans and a proactive approach to future crises. Even though the CPA is now standard practice in UK mental health services, it is not prescriptive about the extent to which there should be consideration of potential failure. There is great variation in the extent to which CPA meetings consider violence risk, and the extent to which they engage in contingency planning. The explicit scenarios of violence as the feared outcome in the HCR20 (Historical Clinical Risk-20) are an example of preoccupation with failure, so it is not surprising that some organizations have adopted it as a standard measure.

The other aspects of a preoccupation with failure are a willingness to acknowledge 'near misses' and learn from them, and the avoidance of blame. They go together because staff who fear blame will be reluctant to acknowledge near misses or errors that may have contributed to them. Weick and Sutcliffe (2001) cite the example of an engineer on a nuclear aircraft carrier, commended for reporting the loss of one of his tools (the risk being that it would be sucked into a jet engine and cause an explosion). Mental health services in the UK are a world away from this culture of safety first.

## Reluctance to simplify

The principle here is that simplification inevitably involves a loss of information, and that information may be critical in avoiding disaster. There are obvious implications for mental health services, which are prone to sacrifice quality in pursuit of higher turnover. If we treat a patient as a generic case of schizophrenia we may not pay sufficient attention to the aspects that make the case unique, such as substance misuse or relationship difficulties. A full risk assessment is multidimensional, so it is of lower quality if we discard information relating to any one dimension.

Similarly, the management of serious risk in psychiatry requires the use of collateral information rather than relying on the patient's account alone. Many homicide Inquiries have commented on the necessity of listening to relations or carers, who often become aware of deterioration in the mental state at a much earlier stage than professionals.

There is a tension here between efficiency and safety. Simplification saves time, effort, and money, while increasing risk. There are political decisions to be made, about the level of risk we can afford to pay for.

## Sensitivity to operations

The principle here is that awareness of detail on the ground is more useful than a strategic overview; the devil is in the detail. On the aircraft carrier, danger lies in a discarded spanner, rather than any more sophisticated problem.

Again, it is easy to find resonances within mental health. Several homicide Inquiries found that the outcome hinged on failures to follow basic, mundane policies such as searching patients after unauthorised absence. Many more revolve around failures of communication, which meant that key facts were not known to the people who could have acted on them. Successful management of violence risk may require an intimate knowledge of the patient's day-to-day life, using as many sources of information as possible. As with the reluctance to simplify, the concern with operational detail implies extra expense.

## Commitment to resilience

Resilience refers to the capacity to plan for untoward events, and it requires that an organization is not working at full stretch. For example, an urgent consultation is only possible if mental health workers have spaces in their diaries. If there is no emergency, the spare slot goes to waste. On the other hand, if there are no spare slots, it is impossible to respond promptly when things go wrong.

There may be duplication of some aspects of the service. The airline pays a second pilot, in case the first has a heart attack. How many mental health services can afford to provide full cover for annual leave? Yet again, there are resource implications.

## Deference to expertise

In a service where many decisions depend on technical expertise, it is essential that the management hierarchy is flexible enough to make use of that expertise. If the technicians advise a particular course of action, it is irresponsible of managers to overrule that advice because it comes from somebody who is low in the pecking order.

When this principle is applied to mental health, it translates easily into a respect for clinical opinion. So when the clinicians advise that violence risk in a particular case can only be safely managed by admission, a manager will think carefully before ignoring that advice. In fact, mental health services do well against this standard, and it is unusual to hear of clinical advice being overruled. A more common problem is that the clinicians know that resources are stretched so they change their recommendation to fit what they know is available. Principle no. 8 above warns against this practice, which is incompatible with a high risk organization.

## Towards a safer service

We may not work in High Reliability Organizations but we can learn from their methods. Clinicians need to take a lead in violence risk management, and to demand from their managers the changes necessary to support safer practice. The opposite has been happening in many UK hospitals. Clinicians have opted out of violence risk management and managers, fearing litigation, have been forced to fill the vacuum with untested risk checklists. Clinicians need to regain the initiative and to shape sensible, effective clinical policies.

In the world beyond our services, all societies are becoming more averse to risk, and there is a hardening of attitudes towards violent offenders. The change is real, and it is worth bearing in mind that when the present Mental Health Act was introduced in England and Wales in 1983, the world was a very different place. Violence risk was not a big political issue, and it was hardly an issue at all within mental health. The orthodox teaching at that time was that there was no statistical association between schizophrenia and violence. The profession knows better now, and the media are alert to any perceived threat of violence to the public, particularly when it is associated with mental disorder.

There are no grounds for optimism that mental health services will be relieved from the ever-growing pressure to reduce violence risk. Public expectations are a fact of life and services have to live with them. Public fears of violence by the mentally disordered may be exaggerated but they are real. Emotions are facts. Public fears must be acknowledged and addressed. In order to retain public confidence the profession needs to demonstrate better risk management skills.

At the same time, we need to educate politicians and the public to have realistic expectations. Not all violence by the mentally ill is preventable, and the overall threat is small compared to violence with other causes. The process of creating realistic expectations involves sharing the risk of violence with other agencies. It also requires a recognition that decisions on the acceptability of risk are not medical matters and ought to be taken by courts or Tribunals whenever possible. The best hope for relief from unreasonable responsibility for violence risk lies in giving up unreasonable power, or sharing it with bodies such as Multi-Agency Public Protection Panels.

The search for better ways of managing violence risk needs to guard against two tempting but false hopes. The first is that actuarial assessment will replace clinical judgement and allow us to know the unknowable. It will not, and we should keep actuarial methods firmly in their place as tools to assist the clinician.

The second unrealistic hope is that capacity- or competency-based legislation will allow us to opt out of the risk assessment business. The case against that possibility has been set out in detail already, but I would like to end by inviting comparison between risk-based services in the UK and competency-based services in the USA. The UK emerges well from that comparison, particularly with regard to the most marginalized and vulnerable patients.

That comparison should also reassure those who worry that risk management is somehow illiberal, and relegates patients' interest to second place in service of the state. There is something shocking about the draconian, 99-year prison sentences imposed on some mentally ill offenders in the USA. They serve as a reminder that the state has its own methods of protecting its citizens from violence. Recent controversy in the UK has raised the spectre of a Government determined to turn mental health services into agents of social control. The USA reminds us that the state has its own methods of social control. The Government does not need psychiatrists to manage violence risk in the mentally ill—but our patients do.

# References

Andrews DA and Bonta, J. (1995) *The Level of Supervision Inventory–Revised*. Toronto, Canada: Multi-Health Systems Inc.

Angermeyer MC (2000) Schizophrenia and violence. *Acta Psychiatrica Scandinavica* 102: 63.

Appelbaum, PS, Robbins PC and Monahan J (2000) Violence and delusions: data from the MacArthur Violence Risk Assessment Study. *American Journal of Psychiatry* 157: 566–572.

Appleby L, Shaw J, Amos T, McDonnell R, Harris C, McCann K, Bickley H, Parsons R, Kiernan K and Davies S (1999) *Safer Services. Report of the National Confidential Inquiry into Suicide and Homicide by People with Mental Illness* London: Stationery Office.

Appleby L, Shaw J, Sherratt J, Amos T, Robinson J, McDonnell R, McCann K, Parsons R, Burns J, Bickley H, Kiernan K, Wren J, Hunt I, Davies S and Harris C (2001) *Safety First. Report of the National Confidential Inquiry into Suicide and Homicide by People with Mental Illness* London: Stationery Office.

Arsenault L, Caspi A, Moffitt TE, Taylor PJ, and Silva PA (2000) Mental disorders and violence in a total birth cohort. *Archives of General Psychiatry* 57: 979–986.

Barraclough BM, Bunch J, Nelson B and Sainsbury P (1974) A hundred cases of suicide: clinical aspects. *British Journal of Psychiatry* 125: 355–373.

Beales DM (2005) eLetter to Psychiatric Bulletin in response to Maden (2005) http://pb.rcpsych.org/cgi/eletters/29/4/121.

Blom-Cooper L, Hally H and Murphy E (1995) *The Falling Shadow. One patient's mental health care*. London: Duckworth.

Blom-Cooper L, Grounds A, Guinan P, Parker A and Taylor M. (1996) *The Case of Jason Mitchell: Report of the Independent Panel of Inquiry*. London: Duckworth.

Bonta J, Law M and Hanson K (1998) The prediction of criminal and violent recidivism among mentally disordered offenders: a meta-analysis. *Psychological Bulletin* 123: 123–142.

Borum R, Bartel P and Forth A (2002) *Manual for the Structured Assessment of Violence Risk in Youth (SAVRY)*. San Diego: Specialised Training Services. See also: www.fmhi.usf.edu/mhlp/savry/statement.htm.

Brennan PA, Mednick SA, Hodgins S. (2000) Major Mental Disorders and Criminal Violence in a Danish Birth Cohort. *Archives of General Psychiatry* 57: 494–500.

Bristol Royal Infirmary Inquiry (2001) *Learning from Bristol: the report of the public inquiry into children's heart surgery at the Bristol Royal Infirmary 1984-1995*. Command Paper: CM 5207.

Buchanan A (1997) The investigation of acting on delusions as a tool for assessing risk and dangerousness. *British Journal of Psychiatry* 170 (Suppl. 32): 12–16.

Buchanan A, Reed A, Wessely S, Garety P and Taylor PJ, Grubin D and Dunn G (1993) Acting on Delusions II: The phenomenological correlates of acting on delusions. *British Journal of Psychiatry* 163: 77–81.

Cheung P, Schweitzer I, Crowley K and Tuckwell V (1997) Violence in schizophrenia: role of hallucinations and delusions. *Schizophrenia Research* 26: 181–190.

Cocozza J and Steadman H (1976) The failure of psychiatric predictions of dangerousness: clear and convincing evidence. *Rutgers Law Review* 29: 1084–1101.

Cooke D (2000) Current Risk Assessment instruments in *A Report of the Committee on Serious Violent and Sexual Offenders (The MacLean Committee)*. Edinburgh: The Scottish Executive.

Cooke D, Michie C and Ryan J (2001) *Evaluating Risk for Violence: A Preliminary Study of the HCR-20, PCL-R and VRAG in a Scottish Prison Sample*. Edinburgh: Scottish Prison Service Occasional Paper 5/2001.

Copas J and Marshall P (1998) The offender group reconviction scale: a statistical reconviction score for use by probation officers. *Applied Statistics* 47: 159–171.

Dawson J and Szmukler G (2006) Fusion of mental health and incapacity legislation. *British Journal of Psychiatry* 188: 504–509.

Department of Health (1994) *Guidance on the Discharge of Mentally Disordered People and their Continuity of Care in the Community*. HSG (94) 27. London: NHS Executive.

Department of Health (1999) *A National Service Framework for Mental Health*. London: Department of Health.

Department of Health and Social Security (1988) *Report of the Committee of Inquiry into the Care and Treatment of Miss Sharon Campbell*. Cmnd 440 London: HMSO.

Dolan M and Doyle M (2000) Violence risk prediction: clinical and actuarial measures and the role of the psychopathy checklist. *British Journal of Psychiatry* 177: 303–311.

Eldergill A (1998) *The Falling Shadow Report and the Deteriorating Patient. Mental Health Act Commission Legal and Ethical Special Interest Group Discussion Paper*. London: Mental Health Act Commission.

Forth AE, Kosson DS and Hare RD (2003) *Hare Psychopathy Check List—Youth Version (PCL-YV) Manual*. Toronto: Multi-Health Systems.

Foucault M (1967) Madness and Civilization – A history of insanity in the age of reason. London: Tavistock.

Foucault M (2001) *Madness and Civilization*. London: Routledge.

Fresan A, Apiquian R, de la Fuente-Sandoval C, Garcia-Anaya M, Loyzaga C and Nicolini H (2004) Premorbid adjustment and violent behaviour in schizophrenic patients. *Schizophrenia Research* 69: 143–148.

Gje X, Brent Donellan M and Wenk E (2003) Differences in personality and patterns of recidivism between early starters and other serious male offenders. *Journal of the American Academy of Psychiatry and the Law* 31: 68–77.

Goldberg D (2005) The narrative and the bureaucratic: an analysis of an independent inquiry report into homicide. *Journal of Forensic Psychiatry and Psychology* 16: 149–166.

Gosden NP, Kramp P, Gabrielsen G, Andersen TF, Sestoft D (2005) Violence in young criminals predicts schizophrenia: a nine year register-based follow-up of 15–19 year old criminals *Schizophrenia Bulletin* 31: 759–768.

Greenwell J, Procter A and Jones A (1997) *Report of the Inquiry into the Treatment and Care of Gilbert Kopernick-Steckel*. Croydon: Croydon Health Authority.

Gunn J (1993) Dangerousness. In Gunn J and Taylor PJ (eds) *Forensic Psychiatry. Clinical, legal and ethical issues*. London: Butterworth Heinemann, pp. 624–645.

Hafner H and Boker W (1982) *Crimes of Violence by Mentally Abnormal Offenders. A psychiatric and epidemiological study in the Federal German Republic*. Cambridge: Cambridge University Press.

Hanson RK (1997) *The Development of a Brief Actuarial Risk Scale for Sexual Offender Recidivism*. User Report 1997–04, Ottawa, Canada: Department of the Solicitor General of Canada.

Hanson RK and Thornton DM (1999) *Static 99: Improving Actuarial Risk Assessments for Sex Offenders*. Ottawa, Canada: Public Works and Government Services Canada.

Hanson RK and Thornton DM (2000) Improving risk assessments for sex offenders: a comparison of three actuarial scales. *Law and Human Behaviour*, 24: 119–136.

Harding TW and Montandon C (1993) 'Does dangerousness travel well?' in Hamilton JR and Freeman H (eds), *Dangerousness: Psychiatric Assessment and Management*. London: Gaskell.

Hare RD (1991) *The Psychopathy Checklist Revised*. Toronto: Multi-Heatlh Systems.

Hare RD (2003) *Hare Psychopathy Checklist-Revised (PCL-R)*, (2nd edn). Technical manual. North Tonawanda, NY: Multi-Health Systems.

Harris GT, Rice ME and Quinsey VL (1993) Violent recidivism of mentally disordered offenders: the development of a statistical prediction instrument. *Criminal Justice and Behaviour* 20: 315–335.

Harris A, Phenix A, Hanson RK and Thornton D (2003) *Static 99 Coding Rules—Revised*. Ottawa: Corrections Directorate, Solicitor General of Canada (www.sgc.gc.ca).

Hart S, Cox D & Hare R (1995) *The Hare Psychopathy Checklist: Screening Version*. Toronto: Multi-Health Systems.

Hart SD (1998) 'Psychopathy and risk for violence' in Cooke DJ, Forth AE and Hare RD (eds), *Psychopathy: Theory, Research and Implications for Society*. Dordrecht: Kluwer, pp. 355–375.

Hawton K, Appleby L, Platt S, Foster T, Cooper J, Malmberg A and Simkin S (1998) The psychological autopsy approach to studying suicide: a review of methodological issues. *Journal of Affective Disorders* 50: 269–276.

Higgins N, Watts D, Bindman J, Slade M and Thornicroft G (2005) Assessing violence risk in adult psychiatry. *Psychiatric Bulletin* 29: 131–133.

Hodgins S (1992) Mental disorder, intellectual deficiency, and crime. Evidence from a birth cohort. *Archives of General Psychiatry* 49: 476–483.

Hodgins S and Muller-Isberner R (2004) Preventing crime by people with schizophrenic disorders: The role of psychiatric services. *British Journal of Psychiatry* 185: 245–50.

Hodgins S, Mednick SA, Brennan PA, Schulsinger F and Engberg M. (1996) Mental disorder and crime. Evidence from a Danish birth cohort. *Archives of General Psychiatry* 53: 489–496.

Home Office (2001) *Statistical Bulletin: Statistics of mentally disordered offenders 2000*. London: Home Office, Research Development and Statistics Directorate.

Humphreys MS, Johnstone EC, MacMillan JF and Taylor PJ (1992) Dangerous behaviour preceding first admission for schizophrenia. *British Journal of Psychiatry* 161: 501–505.

Illich I (1976) *Limits to medicine: medical nemesis – the expropriation of health*. London: Marion Boyars.

Illich I (2001) *Limits to Medicine: medical nemesis–the expropriation of health*. London: Marion Boyars.

Kemshall H (2002) *Risk Assessment and Management of Serious Violent and Sexual Offenders*. Edinburgh: Scottish Executive Social Research.

Kendler KS, Glazer WM, and Morgenstern H (1983) Dimensions of delusional experience. *Am J Psychiatry* 140: 466–69.

Laajasalo T and Hakkanen H (2001) Offence and offender characteristics among two groups of Finnish homicide offenders with schizophrenia: comparison of early- and late-start offenders. *Journal of Forensic Psychiatry and Psychology* 16: 41–59.

Laing RD (1970) *The Divided Self. An Existential Study in Sanity and Madness*. New York: Random House.

Lidz CW, Mulvey EP and Gardner W (1993) The accuracy of prediction of violence to others. *Journal of the American Medical Association* 269: 1007–1011.

Lindqvist P and Allebeck P (1990a) Schizophrenia and crime. A longitudinal follow-up of 644 schizophrenics in Stockholm. *British Journal of Psychiatry* 157: 345–350.

Lindqvist P and Allebeck P (1990b) Schizophrenia and assaultive behaviour: the role of drug and alcohol abuse. *Acta Psychiatrica Scandinavica* 82: 191–195.

Link BJ, Andrews D & Cullen F (1992) The violent and illegal behaviour of mental patients reconsidered. *American Sociological Review* 57: 275–292.

Link BJ and Stueve A (1994) 'Psychotic symptoms and violent or illegal behaviour of mental patients compared to community controls' in Monahan J and Steadman HJ (eds), *Violence and Mental Disorder: Developments in Risk Assessment*. Chicago, IL: University of Chicago Press, pp. 137–159.

Link BJ, Stueve A and Phelan J (1998) Psychotic symptoms and violent behaviours: probing the components of 'threat/control-override' symptoms. *Social Psychiatry and Psychiatric Epidemiology* 33: 55–60.

Link BJ, Monahan J, Stueve A and Cullen FT (1999) Real in their consequences; a sociological approach to understanding the association between psychotic symptoms and violence. *American Sociological Review* 64: 316–322.

Maden A (1999) Review of Blom-Cooper *et al.* (1996), The Case of Jason Mitchell: Report of the Independent Panel of Inquiry; Peay (1996) Inquiries after Homicide; and Greenwell et al (1997) Report of the Inquiry into the Treatment and Care of Gilbert Kopernick-Steckel. *Psychological Medicine* 29 (6) November 1999, pp 1467–1480.

Maden A (2004) Violence, mental disorder and public protection. *Psychiatry* 3 (11): 1–4.

Maden A (2005) Violence risk assessment: the question is not whether but how. *Psychiatric Bulletin* 29: 121–122.

Maudsley H (1874) Responsibility and mental disease. New York: Appleton.

McIvor G, Moodie K, Perrott S and Spencer F (2001) *The Relative Effectiveness of Risk Assessment Instruments. Social Work Research Findings No. 40*. Edinburgh: Scottish Executive Central Research Unit. www.scotland.gov.uk/cru.

Miller WR and Rollnick S (1991) *Motivational Interviewing: Preparing People to Change Addictive Behaviour*. London: Guilford Press.

Moffitt TE (1993) Adolescence-limited and life-course-persistent antisocial behaviour: a developmental taxonomy. *Psychological Review* 100: 674–701.

Mogg A and Bartlett A (2005) Refusal of treatment in a patient with fluctuating capacity—theory and practice. *Journal of Forensic Psychiatry and Psychology* 16: 60–69.

Monahan, J (1981) *The Clinical Prediction of Violent Behaviour.* Government Printing Office, Washington DC and National Institute of Mental Health: Rockville MD (Discussed in Gunn 1993).

Monahan J (1992) Mental disorder and violent behaviour: perceptions and evidence. *American Psychologist* April: 511–521.

Monahan J, Bonnie RJ, Appelbaum PS, Hyde PS, Steadman HJ and Swartz MS (2001). Mandated community treatment: beyond outpatient commitment. *Psychiatric Services* 52: 1198–2005.

Monahan J, Steadman HJ, Silver E, Appelbaum PS, Robbins PC, Mulvey EP, Roth LH, Grisso T and Banks S (2001). *Rethinking Risk Assessment. The MacArthur Study of Mental Disorder and Violence.* Oxford: University Press.

Montandon C & Harding T (1984) The reliability of dangerousness assessments: a decision making exercise. *Br J Psychiatry* 1984 144: 149–155.

Moran P and Hodgins S (2004) The correlates of comorbid antisocial personality disorder in schizophrenia. *Schizophrenia Bulletin* 30 (4) 791.

Moran P, Walsh E, Tyrer P, Burns T, Creed F and Fahy T (2003) Impact of comorbid personality disorder on violence in psychosis. *British Journal of Psychiatry* 182–134.

Mullen PE (1997) A reassessment of the link between mental disorder and violent behaviour, and its implications for clinical practice. *Australia and New Zealand Journal of Psychiatry* 31: 3–11.

Mullen PE (2005) Facing up to our responsibilities: Commentary on The Draft Mental Health Bill. *Psychiatric Bulletin* 29: 248–249.

Mullen PE (2006) Schizophrenia and violence: from correlations to preventative strategies. *Advances in Psychiatric Treatment.*

Mullen P, Taylor PJ and Wessely S (1993) 'Psychosis, violence and crime' in Gunn J and Taylor PJ (eds) *Forensic Psychiatry. Clinical, legal and ethical issues.* London: Butterworth Heinemann 329–371.

Munro E (2004) Mental health tragedies: investigating beyond human error. *Journal of Forensic Psychiatry and Psychology* 15: 475–493.

National Institute for Clinical Excellence (2005) *Violence. The short-term management of disturbed/violent behaviour in inpatient psychiatric settings and emergency departments. Clinical Guideline No. 25.* London: National Institute for Clinical Excellence. http://www.nice.org.uk.

Nolan KA, Czobor P, Biman B, Roy BB, Platt MM, Shope CB, Citrome LL and Volavka J (2003) Characteristics of assaultive behavior among psychiatric inpatients. *Psychiatric Services* 54: 1012–1016.

Peay J (1996) *Inquiries after Homicide.* London: Duckworth.

Petch E and Bradley C (1997) Learning the lessons from homicide inquiries: adding insult to injury? *Journal of Forensic Psychiatry* 8: 161–184.

Quinsey V, Harris G, Rice M and Cormier C (1998) *Violent Offenders: appraising and managing risk.* Washington DC: American Psychological Association.

Rice ME, Harris GT & Cormier CA (1992) An evaluation of a maximum security therapeutic community for psychopaths and other mentally disordered offenders. Law and Human Behavior 16: 399–412.

Ritchie J, Dick D and Lingham R (1994) *The Report of the Inquiry into the Care and Treatment of Christopher Clunis*. London: HMSO.

Royal College of Psychiatrists (1991) *Good Medical Practice in the Aftercare of Potentially Violent and Vulnerable Patients Discharged from Inpatient Psychiatric Care*. London: Royal College of Psychiatrists.

Royal College of Psychiatrists (2005) *Psychiatrists and Multi-Agency Public Protection Arrangements: guidelines on representation, participation, confidentiality and information exchange*. London: Royal College of Psychiatrists www.rcpsych.ac.uk/members/currentissues/publicprotection.aspx.

Sarkar S (2003) BMJ Rapid Response 25.2.2003 to Coid J and Maden A (2003): Should psychiatrists protect the public? *British Medical Journal* 326: 406–407.

Shapiro DE (1999). The interpretation of diagnostic tests. *Statistical Methods in Medical Research* 8: 113–134.

Shaw J, Amos T, Hunt IM, Flynn S, Turnbull P, Kapoor N and Appleby L (2004) Mental illness in people who kill strangers: longitudinal study and national clinical survey. *British Medical Journal* 328: 734–737.

Shaw J, Hunt IM, Flynn S, Meehan J, Robinson J, Bickley H, Parsons R, McCann K, Burns J, Amos T, Kapur N and Appleby L (2006) Rates of mental disorder in people convicted of homicide: a national clinical survey. *British Journal of Psychiatry* 188: 143–147.

Sheppard D (1996) *Learning the Lessons* (2nd edn). London: Zito Trust.

Silva JA, Weinstock R and Klein RL (1995) Psychiatric factors associated with dangerous misidentification delusions. *Bulletin of the American Academy of Psychiatry and the Law* 23: 53–61.

Singh SP & Burns T (2006) Race and mental health: there is more to race than racism BMJ 333: 648–651.

Singleton N, Meltzer H, Gatward R, Coid J and Deasy D (1998) *Survey of Psychiatric Morbidity of Prisoners in England and Wales*. London: HMSO.

Steadman HJ (2000) From dangerousness to risk assessment of community violence: taking stock at the turn of the century. *J Am Acad Psychiatry Law* 28:3:265–271.

Steadman H and Cocozza J (1974) *Careers of the Criminally Insane*. Lexington Books: Lexington Mass (discussed in Gunn, 1993).

Steadman H and Keveles C (1972) The community adjustment and criminal activity of the Baxstrom patients: 1966–70. *American Journal of Psychiatry* 129: 304–310.

Steadman HJ, Monahan J, Robbins PC, Applebaum P, Grino T, Klassen D, Mulvey EP and Roth L (1993) 'From dangerousness to risk assessment: implications for appropriate research strategies' in Hodgins S (ed.), *Mental Disorder and Crime*. London: Sage.

Steadman HJ, Mulvey EP, Monahan, J, Robbins PC, Appelbaum PS, Grisso T, Loren H, Roth LH, Silver E (1998) Violence by people discharged from acute psychiatric inpatient facilities and by others in the same neighborhood. *Archives of General Psychiatry* 55: 393–401.

Steinert T, Voellner A and Faust V (1998) Violence and schizophrenia: two types of criminal offenders. *European Journal of Psychiatry* 12: 153–165.

Stevenson J & Goodman R (2001) Association between behaviour at age 3 years and adult criminality. *British Journal of Psychiatry*, 179, 197–202.

Stueve A & Link BJ (1997) Violence and psychiatric disorders: results from and epidemio-logical survey in Israel. *Psychiatric Quarterly* **68**: 327–342.

Swanson JW, Holzer CE, Ganju VK and Jonjo RT (1990) Violence and psychiatric disorder in the community: evidence from the Epidemiologic Catchment Area surveys. *Hospital and Community Psychiatry* **41**: 761–770.

Swanson JW, Borum R, Swartz MS and Monahan J (1996) Psychotic symptoms and disorders and the risk of violent behaviour in the community. *Criminal Behaviour and Mental Health* **6**: 309–329.

Swanson JW, Swartz MS, Borum R, Hiday V, Wagner R and Burns B (2000) Involuntary outpatient commitment and reduction of violent behaviour in persons with severe mental illness. *British Journal of Psychiatry* **176**: 324–331.

Szmukler G (2000) Homicide Inquiries: What sense do they make? *Psychological Bulletin* **24**: 6–10.

Szmukler G (2003) Risk assessment: 'numbers' and 'values'. *Psychiatric Bulletin* **27**: 205–207.

Taylor PJ (1993) Schizophrenia and crime: distinctive patterns in association. Pp 63–85 in Hodgins S (ed.) *Mental Disorder and Crime*. London: Sage.

Taylor PJ, Garety P, Buchanan A, Reed A, Wessely S, Ray K, Dunn G & Grubin D (1994) Delusions and violence. Pp 161–182 in Monahan J & Steadman HJ (eds) *Violence and Mental Disorder: Developments in risk assessment*. Chicago: University of Chicago.

Taylor PJ & Gunn JC (1984) Violence and Psychosis. British Medical Journal, 288: 1945–9.

Taylor PJ and Gunn J (1999) Homicides by people with mental illness: myth and reality. *British Journal of Psychiatry* **174**: 9–14.

Taylor, R. (1999). Predicting reconvictions for sexual and violent offences using the revised offender group Reconviction scale. *Home Office Research Findings No.104*. London: Home Office.

Teplin LA, Abram KM and McClelland GM (1994) Does psychiatric disorder predict violent crime among released jail detainees? A six-year longitudinal study. *American Psychologist* **49**: 335–342.

Tidmarsh D (1997) Psychiatric risk, safety cultures and homicide inquiries. *Journal of Forensic Psychiatry* **8**: 138–151.

Tihonen J, Isohanni M, Rasanen P, Koiranen M, Morning J (1997) Specific major mental disorders and criminality: a 26 year prospective study of the 1966 Northern Finland birth cohort. *American Journal of Psychiatry* **154**: 840–845.

Tyrer, P. (2000) Personality Assessment Schedule: PAS–I (ICD–10 version). In *Personality Disorders: Diagnosis, Management and Course* (ed. P. Tyrer), pp. 160–180. London: Arnold.

Walsh E, Buchanan A and Fahy T (2002) Violence and shizophrenia: examining the evidence. *British Journal of Psychiatry* **180**: 490–495.

Webster CD, Harris GT, Rice ME, Cormier C and Quinsey VL (1994) *The Violence Prediction Scheme: assessing dangerousness in high risk men*. Toronto, Canada: University of Toronto Centre for Criminology.

Webster CD, Douglas KS, Eaves D and Hart SD (1997) *HCR-20. Assessing Risk for Violence, Version 2*. Vancouver: Mental Health, Law and Policy Institute, Simon Fraser University.

Weick K and Sutcliffe K (2001) *Managing the Unexpected: assuring high performance in an age of complexity*. Michigan: Jossey Bass Wiley.

Wessely S, Buchanan A, Reed A, Cutting J, Everitt B, Garety P and Taylor PJ (1993) Acting on Delusions I: prevalence. *British Journal of Psychiatry* 163: 69–76.

Winterton R (2004) Memorandum of Evidence to Joint Committee on the Draft Mental Health Bill (DMH 396) www.publications.parliament.uk/pa/jt200405/jtselect/jtment/79/5011902.htm.

Wong S, Gordon A (2000) Violence Risk Scale, Version 2. Unpublished. Distributed from Research Unit, Regional Psychiatric Centre, Saskatoon, Canada.

## Law Reports

Re C, 1994 (Adult: refusal of treatment) 1994 1 WLR 290.

# Index